SICKNESS

CAUSES & SOLUTIONS

BY SHANE BLACKBURN

Disclaimer

Diamond Publications and the author are not dispensing medic advice but are offering information of a general nature to help you cooperate with your doctor in your search for better health. Should you use any of the information in this book for yourself, which is yc right, the author or Diamond Publications assume no responsibility for your action. This information presented herein is in no way intended as a substitute for medical counseling. The purpose of thi book is to educate.

Published by:
    Shane Blackburn
    P.O. Box 95
    Hicksville, Ohio 43526

ISBN 0-9766956-3-4

SICKNESS:
CAUSES & SOLUTIONS

CONTENTS

Acknowledgements

To my girl friend Susie (she is also my wife and best friend) who assumed an extra work-load allowing me the time to work on this project. Her continual encouragement and support kept me going.

No book would ever be written without the help of many people. I would like to extend a deep gratitude to the late David Paul Ebaugh of the David Ebaugh Bible School. He understood how I made the connection between the Tabernacle Moses built and the human body. His influence in this project went way beyond encouraging me because I can honestly say he lovingly leaned on me until I committed to put this in manuscript form. Had it not been for him this book would have never been undertaken.

Last, but not least, I want to thank Our Savior who made this all possible.

In regards to body chemistry and health I am indebted to many people who have contributed to my knowledge in this area of my life, and some of them are listed at the end of the book. There are many people who have committed their lives so mankind may have a higher quality of life and we can never repay them for it. We are forever indebted to them.

FOREWARD

Mankind was created by the Almighty with some specific needs for the body, soul, and spirit.

I feel confident any reader will find many answers to questions they have had regarding all three areas mentioned. Shane and Susie are very committed to their nutritional business and are equally committed to this task. Those who read and follow what is written will always be grateful for their diligence.

This book will leave Shane's imprint on many lives. He writes with great interest so clearly and concisely to challenge the reader to live life to its fullest. This masterpiece is a "labor of love" which God has directed and used the author in such a way that will change lives and bring honor to Him.

Jesus said in Matt 25:40 "Verily I say unto you, Inasmuch as ye have done it unto one of the least of these my brethren, ye have done it unto me."

It is the duty of each one of us to learn helpful information and pass it on to others. They have taken this duty seriously.

Dr. Harold Lovelace
Saraland, Al.

INTRODUCTION

In my dealings with people in the area of health over the last 20 years there have been many people who have encouraged me to write a book to share with others what I tell people when I am one-on-one with them in my nutritional business. I am not a medical doctor nor do you need to be one to understand this. You do not have to be a rocket scientist either but you do have to have an open mind and heart. I have endeavored to write this in laymen's terms and for this reason you will not find any complicated medical terms.

There are numerous books on the market in the areas of health and nutrition so it is not my intent to duplicate their efforts.

If a person wants to know the truth regarding any subject, one of the first things they must do is look and see where the masses are in their understanding of said subject. It does not make any difference if you are talking about health, economics, politics or whatever; if the herd is going south you had better be going north, because sheep are always getting sheared. What you are about to read is different than anything you ever read before, and only those who are not afraid to step out of the box will be able to apply these principles to their lives. Most people have the mistaken notion the First Amendment gives us the right to free speech but this is a fallacy. Free speech only applies to accepted or approved thought. It is your right to believe or not to believe what we are sharing with you. It is also your right to apply these principles to your life.

My purpose is to show how we are a three-part person: spirit, soul and body.

It never ceases to amaze me how many sick and unhappy people there are. In America alone we have spent hundreds of billions of dollars over the last 25 years on cancer research, yet this dreaded disease is worse today than ever before. Estimates are by the year 2010 one out of every two Americans will get cancer. We are constantly bombarded by the news media that early detection is the best thing for your chances to beat this to dreaded disease. Knowing you have the disease in its early stages has nothing to do with what is needed so you will never get it in the first place. The same principle applies to heart problems and also to our marriages. The divorce rate in America is currently around 50%. Couples get dressed up and take their vows expecting a happy and fulfilled life. For the marriages that fail those couples find themselves living in a state of unhappiness, in a tired body, and most the time living in an anxious state (if you can call that living).

If you are in poor health or know someone who is, then these principles will interest you. If you are an unhappy person or are in an unpleasant relationship or know someone who is then these principles might interest you also. These principles are for everyone, but this does not mean everyone wants to use them. The only people who are interested in learning these principles are those who desire something better and are willing to take responsibility for them. They then can apply these principles to their lives so they do not end up on the negative side of statistics. If I do not have life abundant, then what do I have, or what am I doing, or what do I need so I can have what my Heavenly Father tells me in His word that He wants me to have: life abundant. This is what I want and if you want it also then these principles will mean more to you.

There is seemingly no reason to search out any alternate health options as long as you think you feel healthy: however, once you are faced with a life threatening situation medical science cannot solve then life takes on a new perspective. At that point if you are a freethinking person you know your present knowledge and value system is inadequate. History shows us there are three personality traits common among people who beat the odds against debilitating diseases: (1) they are fighters, (2) they will make any changes in their life that is necessary, and (3) they must have a spiritual bank to draw on and replace withdrawals on a daily basis. No one can change your value system except you, and if you are not willing to change yours, then the chances of regaining health become much slimmer.
If we want to have a better life than we now have, we must understand why we have the life we do. This will begin to unfold as we get into the upcoming chapters.

Chapter 1
IN THE BEGINNING

To understand why people are physically sick or have emotional instability we have to have the correct understanding of who we are so we can have a better idea of what needs to improve for our life to be changed for the better. God tells us in His word that He created us in His image (Gen 1:26). This means He imaged Himself in us. **We are created as a visible expression of the invisible God. This has not changed. What has changed is our perception of us as a result of the fall.**

> **Num 16:22** says that God is the spirits of all flesh.

> **Zech 12:1** tells us God formed the spirit of man within.

> **Eph 1:4-9** says that He promised us eternal life before the world began. How could He have promised us that if we were not there with Him?

> **John 3:6** says that which is born of the flesh is flesh, and that which is born of the Spirit is spirit. According to Jesus our earthly parents are the parents only of our flesh; for that which was born of the flesh is flesh. Each kind produces after its own kind; cattle beget cattle, dogs beget dogs, etc. God is Spirit so He cannot beget anything but Spirit. He is the Father of spirits.

> **Matt 23:9** says for One is your Father which is in heaven. Until we can see with our minds eye who our Father really is, we will remain in the darkness of our carnal mind. Our dad is not the one who gave us our life that was in the womb of our earthly mother. Once we can recognize that our life did not begin with our physical birth, but it began in heaven, we will have a clearer picture of where to begin making the changes for us to have a more abundant life. Once we recognize where our true heritage exists then we will be less inclined to blame our present situations and conditions on the heritage we thought was ours. Once we become less inclined to blame our families for our present conditions, we will be in a better position to make better decisions to change our situations, which more often than not, we have created for ourselves.

The majority of people fail to reach their goals or obtain a better life for themselves because they make a mental consent to improve or change. One may decide to be a better parent or spouse, a better employee or decide to give up some vice like smoking, drinking, etc. Making a commitment to quit smoking is wonderful, but the problem is as soon as some pressure comes against the smoker the search for the pack is imminent. It is wonderful to make a commitment to be a more thoughtful or considerate spouse but again as soon as your spouse attacks you then you attack back, which leaves both parties being wounded.

There are hundreds of books on the market regarding self-help. That is the problem; they deal with only helping self. These help to a point but until the nature of self is changed there is a limit our mental consent can attain. **We will never reach our potential until our self-nature is changed.**

Our spirit, who we are, is supposed to control our soul (our mind, will, intellect, and emotions) and then our soul is supposed to control our body. Unfortunately, this is not the way most people function. When the soul is in charge then every time we get hurt without going through a healing, the body produces the ill effects we know as being tired, depressed, sick, or diseased.

It is imperative to lock in this thought: our body only does what it is told to do. When the soul signals less destructive thoughts to the body then the body will be given an opportunity to heal. We have no choice in this: every negative thought we have whether it comes from anger, jealousy, envy, resentment, etc., every cell in the body gets flooded with poison. We also can have kindness, gentleness, calmness, and love etc. and when we do, every cell in the body gets a spark of life. **Which ones we have are determined by the choices we make which are determined by our attitudes. The soul is the battleground of conflicting thought, conflicting desire, and conflicting emotions. It is our soul that thinks, not our brain. The brain is the conduit that channels what goes on within our soul.** To illustrate this, we all have heard or read accounts of people who had died, and experienced themselves leaving their body. Whether they saw their bodies lying on an operating table, or at the scene of an accident, where is their brain? It is still in the body they are looking at. They are still experiencing these various thoughts while outside of the body yet their brain is still in the body. Again, it is the soul that thinks, not our brain.

After the fall man has hidden from himself, and in doing so is living totally in the physical world. By doing so man lives in a materialistic world and materialism strips a person of his/her need to feel responsible for themselves and their actions. It is unfortunate but in many cases religion is used for the same reason. If you have a desire to change your attitudes you must first see the battleground going on between the soul and spirit.

In the Garden, man was created to be led by the spirit (the inner man), but after the fall the soul became dominant. When the soul (our mind, will, intellect, and emotions) is dominant then our decisions are made not on the basis of what God would say in our spirit, but on the basis of what we decide based on what we see, hear, taste, smell, and feel. A person who is led from outside influences is a soulish person, but a person who is led from deep within is a spiritual person. We all know people who are totally controlled by their circumstances because they only make decisions using their five physical senses and their lives are emotional wrecks. This then leads to their physical body breaking down into the various diseases. If we would like to live a life that is free from anxiety, depression, frustrations, etc. in a body that is healthy and ready to go at all times, then we must learn to reverse the life we have lived that created our present situations and conditions. If we want to rise above our present circumstances we have to change our perception of ourselves. If we want to make a better life for ourselves then we are the one responsible for the changes that must be made. People have a standard they live by which is someone else's standard. How many of us think we have failed as a mate, parent, employee or employer, etc.? The reason we do this is because of the image we have of ourselves which is based on our past failures and sins. Negative people constantly think of past failures, but positive people constantly think of past successes. When we begin to see ourselves as God sees us instead of how man has programmed us to see ourselves, then we will be in a position to start making positive changes in our lives.

Keep in mind that for us to regain our health and happiness we must understand how and why we have poor health and unhappiness in our soul first.

Any child who ever went to Sunday school knows the story of Sodom and Gomorrah. The angel told Lot to tell his family not to look back once they left. As you know Lot's wife did turn back and God turned her into a pillar of salt. Unfortunately, this same scene is played out every day on this earth. Women who have ever canned know that salt is a preservative. What God did was pickle that woman in her past. People today who continually want to talk about their past, whether it is about someone who did something to them or did not do something for them, are never free to enjoy life today. They lose so much time and energy spent in the past where they are kept prisoners that they are not free to see the love that is in their life today. Their entire life is spent seeing people and circumstances through the child that has been injured. They live their entire life in the dark side of their mind. You can constantly hear them say things like: I will never get that promotion, or I will always be sick, or I'll never have enough money, or if my wife would only do this, or if my husband would not do this and the list goes on. We can never get out of that trap until we begin being thankful and grateful for everything that has ever happened to us and is happening to us today. The human mind can have a dozen thoughts in a second, but it cannot have two at one time. We cannot have negative thoughts of our past when we are living in a state of being grateful today. Only by living in this day we have been given will we be able to grow into a richer and fuller life. The darker mind that most people live in robs them of the riches they were intended to enjoy.

We must be responsible for establishing and maintaining our health because the medical community only assumes responsibility for us after we get sick. When we

3

(the spirit man) gets sick (and we have not learned how to read this language) then our emotions go astray. When our emotions go astray, and we have not learned how to read this language either, then our bodies will develop problems as a result. The medical community is like a child who does not know how to read but picks up a book and starts jabbering away. When doctors are pouring chemicals into a patient or are cutting something out of them they are trying to convince us they know how to read. There are many good caring doctors in the medical community and I am grateful for them because we need them. If someone gets in an accident we need someone to patch him or her up, or if someone is having a heart attack then I am grateful for those who have been trained to try and spare their life.

They have not been trained to teach us how to avoid developing heart problems, cancer, diabetes and other threatening diseases. Their training is geared for after the fact. It is our intent to teach you how to read the language in yourself and your loved ones. If you do, the benefits will last you a lifetime and beyond for your children and grandchildren.

God has laid out a program for us to follow and when we do we will see and understand what He is doing to help us live a better life. Even when we just begin to see what He has planned for us, we will have a greater hope in today and in our future than we ever dreamed of before. There are two things that our Father wants to have placed in our heart: one is hope and the other is mercy. Both of these will be unfolded as we follow the pattern that He laid out for us.

Look at the lady in the picture. There is so much darkness that it is nearly impossible to see any light in her at all with natural eyes. Only with the eyes of Christ can you truly see her as she really is: in His image. She obviously does not know where she came from, why she is here, nor has any hope of having anything better, either in this life or in the one to come. It is only by experiencing the principles we are going to outline in the upcoming chapters will she be able to have a better life than she now has.

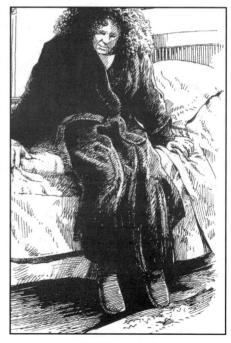

CHAPTER 2
SEEING THE PROTOTYPE

Look at the two pictures below and we are going to discuss in the upcoming chapters how the picture of the man is hidden in the picture of the Tabernacle.

The Structure and Dimensions of the Tabernacle

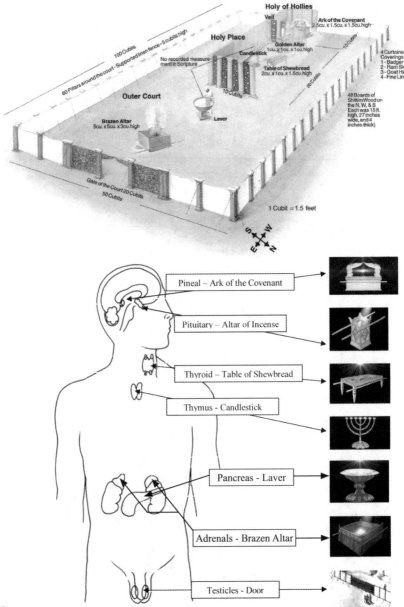

The Tabernacle had three sections in it but there were seven positions where the priest ministered. We must see ourselves in the Tabernacle because if we cannot apply today what all the rituals meant or pointed to (spiritual realities) then we are left with nothing but a history lesson.

There are three aspects of our life that each location in the Tabernacle pointed to (1) there are spiritual lessons to be incorporated into our nature (this goes beyond our understanding the lessons, they are to become a part of us), (2) which leads us to becoming more emotionally stable, (3) which puts our body in a position where it is more likely to heal. When we learn the three aspects at each of the seven locations, we will have a deeper understanding of how we are a three-part person and we should also have a deeper understanding of how we were wonderfully made and then know how to better take care of ourselves.

The seven steps to Moses Tabernacle which prefigure the human body are as follows (1) the door, (2) the altar, (3) the laver, (4) the lampstand, (5) the table of shewbread, (6) The Golden incense altar and (7) the Ark of the Covenant. This is recorded in the 25th chapter of Exodus.

Here is a brief description of each of them in more detail:

(1) The Door - This allowed entrance in the Tabernacle from the outside world.

(2) The Brazen Altar- The first thing the priest saw when he entered from the outer court. This is where the animals were sacrificed.

(3) The laver (washbasin) - Both the priest and the sacrifices were washed here. The outside and inside of the sacrifices were washed speaking of an outer and inner cleansing in our lives.

(4) The Candlestick (lampstand) - This was seen upon entering the Holy room. Olive oil was the fuel used and the priests trimmed the wicks daily.

(5) The Table of Shewbread- This had 12 pancakes on it, which was made of finely ground flour. This speaks of Him grinding finely His nature into ours.

(6) The Golden Altar of Incense-The sacrifices of prayer and praise were given here.

(7) The Ark of the Covenant- On the top of the ark was the mercy seat. On top of the mercy seat were two cherubim with outstretched wings. A crown of gold was around the ark and the Ark contained a pot of manna, Aaron's rod, and the tablets of the law.

There are numerous books available on the market giving details of how the Tabernacle was constructed and what materials were used along with the different dimensions that explain their spiritual significance. You must be able to see the spiritual significance of the various metals used, the various colors, dimensions, etc. or else the entire description becomes nothing but a history lesson. In our walk through the Tabernacle we are going to confine our attention to the seven areas to learn the spiritual, emotional and physical lessons at each area.

If for any reason we do not follow the same pattern in our daily lives that was laid out in the Tabernacle, then we definitely will not have abundant life. If we still harbor all the negative emotions instilled in us at an early age, then it is a guarantee our family will be void of peace and joy. If one experienced a lot of yelling, backbiting, slandering, jealousy, and hatred in the family, then you know some or all the members are filled with these unresolved conflicts. What you were given as a young person has no bearing on your present life unless you want it that way. Everyone is looking for someone to blame their problems on; but they will not have a peaceful life. You have to mature and make the best of what life is giving you. There is not a man walking that does not have a little boy in him who has not been hurt, and every lady also has a little girl in her that has been hurt. If the little one does not get healed the adult will never reach their potential because it is the little one inside that holds the adult in bondage. What people do not understand is that there is not a human who can heal the little one for you; only God can heal him or her. This is what walking through the Tabernacle is all about. This is why we must follow the same walk in the Tabernacle to have our hearts and minds healed. Today God is still diligently seeking those who love Him who have decided to place themselves on the altar for Him to do the necessary inworking in their lives so He can manifest his glory on the earth through them. Those who complete the walk through the Tabernacle are the ones mentioned as overcomers in Revelations 3:21.

Let us now look at the system of the body that correlates to the Tabernacle, and how it is affected by the various emotions and attitudes. It is impossible for our body to exist without a steady supply of nutrients to sustain us. These nutrients come in the form of food, air and water. The fuel (food, air and water) is converted to energy to feed our cells. When the cells are healthy we know the cells are balanced, and when we are tired, depressed, sick or diseased we know they are not balanced. **The body was created to be a fine tuned piece of machinery and our Heavenly Father put within us a glandular system to help or aid us in maintaining our machine.**

The glandular system is called the endocrine system and is composed of seven glands (there is that number seven again!). The endocrine glands secrete hormones into the bloodstream and have a tremendous effect on the body's functions. These hormones work together with our nervous system to regulate or coordinate the activities necessary for our bodies to be harmonious. The endocrine system helps monitor the different systems we have to determine their respective energy levels or lack of. When it is determined there is something not quite right, various glands start producing hormones to accomplish whatever is necessary to maintain balance and efficiency in our bodies. Each one of the seven glands is connected together and each has a predetermined amount of energy within itself. If one of these glands were to become weakened, then one of the others, or maybe all of them would give up a little of their own energy to the weakened one to maintain or reestablish balance. We will discuss in more detail the seven glands in the upcoming chapters, but for now, we will discuss how our emotions affect them.

A portion of our brain called the hypothalamus is the connecting link between our mind and our body. The hypothalamus can stimulate any gland in the endocrine system to produce hormones to prepare our body for various responses (depending on the circumstances). The hypothalamus responds to stress, either imaginary or real, because this is the section of the brain where thoughts are translated into physiological changes in our body. When we begin to understand we have some control over what we think about, then we can begin to understand we have some control over our health. Whether good or evil comes against us is immaterial to us being ill or having good health, but rather how we respond to what comes against us. Somewhere in the hypothalamus a process occurs that stores or keeps emotionally loaded memory associations. We have the potential to release these associations. If and when we go through forgiveness or releasing certain people who are involved in our bad memories, then we let loose or release locked energies in our bodies. **If we have any locked up bad memories, which translates into locked up energy, then this changes or alters our biochemistry, which robs us of our energy.** In addition, any stored negative memories not only inhibit learning but also make us more susceptible to developing psychosomatic diseases.

Forgiveness is necessary for our health because we can never have total divine health without having experienced total divine forgiveness. Contrary to what most adults think God did not give little children more energy; it is just that little ones are not weighted down with feelings of guilt, shame, anger, resentment, grief, jealousy, etc. They just love, so their biochemistry has not been changed for the worse.

All the negative emotions produce more acid in our bodies, which eventually creates inflammation that leads to pain. We will discuss this in more detail later.

The sooner we learn this fact the better off we will be and this translates into better health. We were created with the ability to see life in only two ways, positive or negative. We have the choice and make it many times on a daily basis. We basically determine the direction our life is going to take. Once we learn that every thought we possess (either positive or negative) finds every cell in our body, and that nothing or anyone of an inferior nature can affect us without our permission, the better our health will be. We were created for love and joy; unfortunately, the masses hardly ever find it. No matter what happens to us, either positive or negative, extracts an attitude from us. What develops in us later is dependent on which attitude we faced it with.

We will never be happy with what we want if we are not happy with what we have. **It is not as important what things we have in this life but how much we enjoy the things we have.**

Most people cannot enjoy the things they have because they live in the dark side of their mind. Some people feel safe and secure with their sicknesses and diseases because they get to control people (go get me this, go get me that, do not go too far in case I need you). What a sad state for these people who choose to have a life such as this. These poor people live in a constant state of fear because they know if they get healed they would have to become responsible for themselves

The only thing we really have is what we have to give away. It does not make a difference if you are two years old or 102. Whenever we take more out of life than we put back we become dissatisfied with our life, become bored, become more prone to depression, and consequently we lose the joy of the life we have been given. It is important to know that we can change our thinking and our attitudes no matter what circumstances we are in because of former choices. We can change our attitudes and begin enjoying what we have instead of having a fairytale world of dreaming things different so we do not continue making the same painful decisions over and over again. Our circumstances will change as we change our attitudes. Remember: experience is not what happens to us; it is what we do with what happens to us.

Our democratic society for years has programmed the masses that they (the people) need them (the government). We (the government) will give you free food, free education, free medical supplies, free spending money; all you (the people) have to do is to what we (the government) say. Then the government grabs you with a hook in your nose and leads you to the Promised Land. People who take unnecessary handouts become servants to their masters. The master tells you how much you can have and basically where you will live. If you have a mindset that you are going to vote in a different master so you will have a land of milk and honey, then no matter how you cut the cake, you will always be the slave to the master. It is a choice!! We can either work or be lazy, and enjoy our work (however menial) or not. What do you want? It is your choice! Even though we make choices the consequences of those choices are already established.

The keys to the kingdom that Peter was given are recorded in II Peter1:5-7, which is another account of a walk through the Tabernacle. Peter is mentioning seven specific attitude changes that must be made in order to enter into perfection. They must be entered one after another but the word perfect does not mean perfect as we know it in the English-language. Growing into perfection means becoming mature sons. The seven steps are as follows;

FAITH
VIRTUE
KNOWLEDGE
SELF-CONTROL
PERSEVERANCE
GODLINESS
BROTHERLY KINDNESS
LOVE

I know this is eight but when you have the attributes of the first seven in your nature you will be one of love. Always remember that God is love; He is not judgment, He is love! There is the judgment side of God, but He is not judgment. Never forget; He is love!

<u>As He walks us to through Tabernacle He grinds each one of these characteristics into our nature. While doing so the corresponding gland in the body will automatically be healthier.</u>

Now let's start at the bottom of our bodies and work up to see how our attitudes and choices affect us physically. Keep in mind that we have our problems or conflicts in our spirit first, then our soul, and finally our body.

If the above personality traits do not become part of our nature then our emotions will always control us and we will never attain stability in our life. Most people never operate beyond their five senses. This is recorded in the parable of the 10 virgins (Matthew 25:1-13). People who are controlled by their five senses are represented today by the five virgins who were not ready. Remember: most people cannot function if they cannot smell it, see it, touch it, hear it, or taste it.

We were taught that our brain controlled everything in our body but today we know this is not the case. Our immune system controls the brain. The endocrine glands produce hormones that give us our zest for life. We will discuss balancing hormones in greater detail in chapter 13. You will notice that young people just married are not sick because their hormones are flying all over the place. Why this changes will give us a better understanding of our health or lack of.

As I said earlier the Tabernacle that Moses built was a pattern for our life. John 1:12 shows us that becoming a Son of God is a progressive walk. Jesus taught us about the seven steps into which we should progress. He lived the steps that are parallel to the types and shadows of the steps in the Old Testament Tabernacle. What God did for us is He picked up this Tabernacle and placed it right in the middle of John's Gospel. In consecutive order starting with chapter 10 to and through John 17, he divides into seven steps that which parallel and interpret the seven steps of Moses' Tabernacle. The upcoming seven chapters outline this for us.

CHAPTER 3
THE DOOR CORRELATES TO THE GONADS

The Door is covered in John Chapter 10. Here is a brief description of the glands the Door represents.

THE TESTES

They are involved in sperm production as well as secretion of testosterone. If the testes begin to weaken the man can have an excessive sex drive. He possibly can have extra body hair and occasionally experience some swelling. If the testes weaken further then infertility can appear along with less sexual motivation and the man usually experiences weaker masculine stature.

THE OVARIES

The ovaries are the woman's counter part to the man's testes. They are involved in ovulation and also in the production of progesterone and estrogen. If they begin to weaken the woman may experience in between period pain and excessive flow. This increases her chances of emotional instability and she may begin having vaginal discharge and begin putting weight on her hips and buttocks. When they become further weakened infertility may result and she will experience less sexual interest and could possibly experience painful menstruation. The ovaries greatly influence her mood swings and general health, partially because around her period she may experience indigestion.

Now let's spiritually look to the counterpart to our gonads (THE DOOR: CHRIST JESUS).

Jesus' life taught the Old Testament experience and we must learn it also if we are going to become kings and priests as recorded in Revelation 1:6.

In John 10:7-10 we are told that any man or any message that brings mankind anything but life is a thief and a robber. All the messages brought before Jesus came, led to death.

In Matthew 22:2-14 Jesus tells a parable concerning a marriage. He said anyone trying to slip into the marriage feast (trying to enter the kingdom) and not having on a white robe would be thrown out. They would be thrown out to show Jesus is the door to Heavenly perfection (the only door). Jesus is the way into the kingdom. Trying to enter through some counterfeit way or truth (like sliding under the flap at the wedding) will get you thrown out. It is sad the perception most people have of our Savior because the only thing they know about Him is what other people have said. We will begin to look at some of these perceptions in the upcoming chapters. For now we will share one of them with you.

Most Christian people believe and teach that if you accept the Lord Jesus Christ as your Savior you will be saved. There is more to it than this. The verse that most Christians use to substantiate their belief is Romans 10:9 and in the KJV version it reads as follows: "That if thou shall confess with thy <u>mouth</u> the Lord Jesus Christ, and shall believe in thine heart that God hath raised Him from the dead thou shall be saved." Using the English language this verse cannot be true as it was translated. If you look at the Strong's concordance the word mouth in this verse was translated from the Greek word stoma (#G4750) and it should read <u>*face*</u>. What a tremendous difference this makes in our understanding. Our face is what is supposed to confess our faith in the Lord Jesus Christ. It is not what we say but what we show. When Jesus took the three disciples up on the mountain their countenance would have glowed; likewise, when we truly experience Him as our Savior our countenance should reflect the same. Most Christians are so judgmental because they skim over the verse in Matthew 7:1: therefore, people outside of the Church never see God's mercy. The Church has put so much more emphasis on the sins of the body vs. sins of the disposition. It is a lot harder to live with the person who nags, whines, complains, and is critical and negative vs. one who is living in bodily sin. You cannot have a critical nature and at the same time have His joy. Without His joy we will look like we just came from a wake, and without His joy we will never make good ambassadors for Him.

When we truly experience in our inner being the reality of what He did at Calvary for us then our demeanor will be totally changed. To know within ourselves that everything that we ever said or did that was wrong is completely forgiven and forgotten by our Heavenly Father has a profound effect on our body. HE will never bring them up again, but our fellow man sure will. When I say our fellow man, this definitely includes us. Remember the entire calamity that fell on Job and his three friends came to him to accuse him of all kind of sins. We all experience the same three friends on a daily basis who accuse us of what we did and their names are: me, myself and I.

It was in God's heart for us to have abundant life, but man tries to keep us in bondage so it will always escape us. To truly know what He did for us will have a profound effect on the value we have of our life. To come to the full realization that we never did anything to secure our redemption and do not have to do anything to keep it removes a heavy burden from us. We have a lot more to jump out of bed for in the morning when we realize He established the value of our life and not man. Remember, we are spirit and He is a quickening spirit; therefore, as we have more life in us then our bodies will have more life in them also. You see, Christ Jesus begins our spiritual life and our testicles begin our physical life.

When couples get married they find their reproductive systems work just fine. They work just great because both people are enjoying something new and exciting, experiencing more freedom, etc. Both parties are giving and are excited about just being together, and each one is an extension of the other. It is like all your fingers and toes extend out and your mate is connected to all of them. Problems begin when one of them says something or does something that hurts or wounds the other partner and the wounded one pulls in one or two of his/her fingers and toes so they cannot get hurt again. Most of the time the one who offended is completely unaware of what happened, and then when one mate withdraws the communication begins to break down.

This hurt may not have been something of a negative manner but it was perceived that way. The husband may be working extra hard (because he loves providing for his wife) and does not see that his wife feels she is taking a backseat to his job. Most of the time children come along and the wife is so busy with her children that the husband begins feeling neglected. It is a real fine line to maintain a proper balance between home and work, but it can be done if this is your priority. Every person's priority should be to put God first (this means to have a relationship with his Son), then your mate, then your children if you have any, then your job, then your Church, and finally your social life. Should the husband have this out of order, then with paying less attention to his wife and her needs she will continue to withdraw additional toes and fingers until they are all drawn in.

She is now feeling isolated from the love she chose and will turn to her next priority, which are her children. Her children now become her main focus or at least above that of her husband. What happens with either or both partners in the relationship having other priorities above their mates is that the romance will dwindle. Even though our gonads are at the bottom of the ladder in our endocrine system they are still the furnace that heats up the rest of the glands in the system; likewise, the same thing happens to us emotionally when our romance dwindles because the other aspects of our relationship dwindle also. What begins to happen is our furnace has less heat in them and we begin to have less health or vitality in our gonads. When we throw less coal in the furnace (our gonads) the rest of the body cools down proportionally.

This all correlates to the parable Jesus gave regarding the farmer sewing his grain. Some seed germinated and began growing but weeds grew up and overpowered them. Spiritually people want to do right but the cares of this material world crowd out our spiritual growth. Emotionally we want good relationships but other priorities direct too much of our time and energies away from developing them.

Let us begin to see how some of these principles play out in our body. Keep in mind that we are spirit, soul, and body. God put in man (spirit) to provide for his family. God creates all life but man makes it. Life comes from the male: that is the reason for the virgin birth. If women gave 50% life then Jesus would have had 50% sin in him. God creates it, man makes it, and women give it. So man produces a life and then goes out and gets a job to produce life for the life that he produces. He works to buy clothes, food, a home and other essentials of life. In his mind this is his responsibility and he will continue doing it for the rest of his life. How many men have worked all their life and then when they are 65 years old are forced to retire, and then die two years later with testicle and/or prostate cancer. You see they had been producing all their life and then man comes along and tells them they no longer can. What happens is the reproduction they had in their heart has been cut out which affects the reproduction in their body. When life is taken out of the heart and mind, it will also be taken out of the body. God is constantly trying to put life in us but man is always trying to take it away!

Let's see how this plays out in the woman. The woman's uterus gives life and their breasts nurture it. God put it in the woman to nurture their family but man comes along and tells them this is insufficient. If any mother feels she has not nurtured her children no matter what else she may accomplish in life, she will never feel fulfilled. So many women have worked very hard in the work force to get ahead. If after all the children are gone any mother who realizes she has missed so much will then greatly increase her chance of breast trouble. How many mothers, and/or grandmothers, have raised their children or grandchildren only to find that they have gone astray? Some of them do not even know where the children or grandchildren are living or if they are living at all. The breasts nurture the life that they gave and now that life has been taken away. The nurturing in the heart is being sucked out; consequently, life potentially will be sucked out of their breasts. I use the word potentially because women will not necessarily develop breast trouble just because they have these losses in life.

This is why it is so important to put our Heavenly Father first in our life because if He is our first love then He will sustain us during these dark times. It is important to know that these tragedies do not have to have a stranglehold on us; unfortunately, this is not the case in most situations. Mastectomies are performed on cancerous breasts hoping that all the cancer has been removed from the body, but the patient in the recovery room still has the pain in her heart that caused the problem in the first place. It is sad that the health-care business in our country is basically a sick-based industry. Not enough time is spent finding out why people are hurt (emotionally) and trying to teach them how to stay healthy. We are told early detection is so important, and it is, but it has nothing to do with why we get the disease in first place.

It is astonishing to think of going to a college football game on Saturday afternoon where there are 100,000 people present and knowing that one out of three people in this country are getting cancer, so 33,000 of those fans have cancer in them and do not even know it yet. Just the thought of it puts fear in most people and rightfully so because no one gives any of them hope of prevention. The emphasis right now is on breast cancer: any mother who has a loving relationship with her husband and her children greatly reduces her chances of future breast cancer. There definitely is more to breast cancer than this because diet and other factors are involved. Some of these will be discussed in a later chapter. Man (by his inherent nature) continually tries to drain us of our life. This cannot happen without our permission.

Our Heavenly Father wants us to have abundant life and unfortunately, most people do not find it. In the upcoming chapters we will see the program He laid out for us in the Tabernacle for us to obtain abundant life. It is such a wonderful thing to know that our sins are forgiven, but there is so much more He wants to give us. Christian people want to talk about what Jesus did for them 2000 years ago (He definitely did) and what He is going to do for us when we die, but most of them seem oblivious to what He is trying to do for us today.

One of the things He plans for us is to put us in a position to make better choices for ourselves. You know the sun falls on wax and clay at the same temperature, but one gets hard and one gets soft; the same principle applies to human hearts. No one is immune from tragedy, adversity, or evil during his or her life, but some become softer and some become harder because of it. The difference is determined by choices or attitudes while going through it. One thing for sure, we were not created to stagnate, and if all you have ever experienced is having your sins forgiven then you are missing one of the greatest blessings of all: TO KNOW HIM! This will begin to unfold in the upcoming chapters.

Knowing Him was Paul's greatest drive in life. The average Christian cannot get to this level of relationship with Him because after the fall in the garden man merely sees himself in a master-slave relationship with Him. God is invisible and the only way to see the attributes of God is in the physical, and the most complete attributes of God are shown in the marriage of the husband and wife. Man's fallen nature has blurred this vision. For the most part, the male sexual experience has been geared toward their gratification at the expense of the woman, while females tend to experience their emotional gratification at the expense of the man.

This is why Christ within walks us through the Tabernacle so the inner conflicts, brought on by being wounded, can be healed. If this does not happen then at best each mate uses the other to make love to him or herself. This is spiritual masturbation. When this happens our life energy is thwarted, which places our gonads (both male and female) in a position to be compromised. This leads them into a variety of maladies. As always, we are sharing this with you so you have a better understanding of cause and effect. Without this understanding, you remain spiritually blind and being spiritually blind interferes with our emotional stability and without emotional stability our health cannot be maintained.

Chapter 4
THE ALTAR CORRELATES TO THE ADRENALS

The altar is covered in chapters 11 and 12 of John's Gospel. They both depict death; Chapter 11 covers the death of Lazarus, and Chapter 12 covers His own death. Death symbolically is connected to our adrenals.

The adrenals produce anti-inflammatory hormones and they regulate water levels in the body. They also are involved in carbohydrate and blood sugar regulation. In addition they are also involved in the body's equilibrium under stress and also are involved in speeding up ones metabolism when under stress.

When these two glands begin to weaken one may become nervous and irritable. Hypertension may begin along with edema. One may begin bruising easily and the stomach may begin sagging. When these glands become further weakened one may experience lack of energy and become dizzy. At this point one may also be more prone to allergies, experience muscle weakness, and become mentally lethargic. A person will also become more prone to depression and will have a harder time getting up in the morning. The adrenals are referred to as our stress glands because under stress they produce so many hormones that without them we would die in a day or so unless we begin hormone replacement.

All of the glands in the endocrine system have primary functions in addition to secondary ones. We mentioned earlier that the testicles produce the male hormone testosterone but a small amount of this hormone is produced by the adrenals. If this hormone is not produced then he becomes frigid. These glands also produce the cortex hormones that keep inflammation in check. This is extremely valuable in cases of inflammatory diseases like arthritis, bursitis, gout, colitis and even asthma. Some patients have pain that is so unbearable that they have to take cortisone based drugs; unfortunately, these drugs weaken the adrenals further causing the bones to weaken which leads to anemia.

To understand why the adrenals get so weakened we must first see them spiritually. Remember we said earlier that after walking through the door of the Tabernacle the first thing you saw was the altar. This was where the animal was killed for the sacrifice. **We will never progress beyond where we are living until we see ourselves in the little animal.** We know that the animal was a prototype of Christ Jesus who was to come later; but remember, Paul said, "I die daily"! Paul says in Phil 1:21 "To die is gain." There is no gain in going to the cemetery, but to die to the carnal mind is to gain the mind of Christ. To die to the natural is to gain the spiritual. To die to the Adam nature is to gain the divine nature. God's people have a mistaken notion this phrase "to die" implies some awful physical death. This is referring to a spiritual growth in Him. *The cross (the cross we must carry) is* *a place of execution. It is the place where our <u>Adam nature</u> reaches its final doom. To teach otherwise is to blasphemy God's word.* Let's look at how this plays out in our physical bodies.

The first emotion that Adam and Eve experienced after the fall was fear (Genesis 3:10). THE ADRENALS ARE DESTROYED BY FEAR! You see everyone wants to go to heaven, but no one wants to die. Far too often people want Jesus to be their Savior because they are afraid of going to hell. He did not die for us on the cross just to get us into heaven but to start us on a journey back to our Father. Christian people want Jesus to be their Savior but they certainly do not want him to be their LORD. They like the idea of going to heaven but they still want to be in control of their life. They want to do what they want to do, when they want to do it. This includes harboring all the negative emotions against anyone and everyone who has ever hurt them or their loved ones. This is one of the main reasons why so many Christians are so judgmental and critical. As long as they can get you focused on your shortcomings and sins then you cannot see all the unresolved conflicts in them.

People do not want to change so they create a God who agrees or is like them. They certainly would not kill someone because they do not want to go to hell, but they sure want Jesus to torture those who have hurt them. Most Christian people are struck with fear at the thought of facing God because He hates sin and cannot tolerate it. Even though they are afraid of Him they know that He will accept them into heaven because His blood covers us. It is a shame that today most Christian people fear God as have all mankind through the centuries. Remember the Hebrew people (after God miraculously led them as they passed through the sea and then continued miraculously feeding them) being petrified to face Him on the mountain because He was a God of thunder and lightning (Exodus 19:16).

The dominant image most Christian people have of their Father is that He will squash them as little ants if they get out of line. It is like they perceive Him hiding in the bushes trying to catch them having some fun. How would we as adults feel if we called one of our children and they came to us trembling because they were afraid of us? It is fine to instill in children that dad will enforce consequences for misconduct, but unless there is any violation or rebellion against clearly outlined rules, the children should never have any fear of their parents. Any loving parent would be devastated if they thought their children were afraid of them; unfortunately, this is how most people feel about our Heavenly Father. In the Old Testament God called Abraham His friend and we will never be His friend as long as we are afraid of Him. This is experiencing the altar in our lives. *We must die to ourselves so everything that has been put in us to keep us from a loving relationship with Him must be removed.* So many Christian people want to die for Jesus but that is not what He wants; what He wants is for us is to live for Him. What a tremendous difference! We cannot live for him in a state of fear. Here are a few versus that shed light on this.

Psalms 32:2 "Blessed is the man to whom the LORD <u>shall not</u> impute sin". Impute means charge his account with.

Romans 4:8 "Blessed is the man to whom the LORD <u>does not</u> impute iniquity"

I Corinthians 1:30 "But of Him you are in Christ Jesus, who became for us wisdom from God-and righteousness and sanctification and redemption." This tells us that we stand righteous before God (He is our righteousness) then there is nothing on our record.

Colossians1:21-22 "He has (past tense) reconciled us to present us holy, blameless and above reproach in His sight." This is how God sees us but man has twisted this so we will view ourselves through our eyes instead of His. As we pointed out earlier most people live in the dark side of their mind. This makes it impossible for them to perceive themselves in any other light. We will never begin growing closer to Him until we perceive ourselves as He perceives us.

If the above versus do not touch us then we will remain living in the dark side of our mind and the chances of having our adrenal glands healed are slim to none. Let's look at a couple of situations that develop in the body when our adrenals are weak.

When the body is in a stressful situation the adrenals are forced to work harder. Let's say you are walking down the street and a man jumps out in front of you with a knife; for most people they are left with two options, either fight him or run from him. This is referred to as the fight or flight syndrome. Regardless of which choice we make the body needs an immediate response to meet our energy needs. The body does this for us in the following manner. The hypothalamus in our brain (some call it a gland) receives messages from our five senses and depending on how the information is interpreted the hypothalamus will instruct the pituitary what needs to be done for us to maintain our balance. This is accomplished through hormones. Our pituitary produces hormones, which are sent down to the other six glands in the system.

Under stress the adrenals are told to produce and release cortisol. Cortisol is the hormone that will elevate the sugar in our blood because sugar is the fuel (energy) we need to either fight or run. Cortisol is produced regardless of whether the stress is physical, mental or emotional. If one has an overpowering boss or husband, a nagging wife or extreme financial burdens, cortisol will be produced. In our society though, we do not run or fight. This then can lead to several health problems. When our life is under constant stress then the adrenals will get exhausted. When this condition develops then levels of cortisol produced will be below normal. This is why people with adrenal fatigue (hypoadrenia) usually end up with low blood sugar (hypoglycemia). Most people, when they develop either of these two conditions, usually start eating more to try to boost their energy levels; unfortunately, they invariably begin putting on weight. This usually occurs around the middle (the spare tire look). Too many people (especially the ladies) at this point try using diet pills.

When the adrenals further weaken then one becomes more prone to allergies, asthma, begin experiencing more frequent colds and respiratory infections and other conditions. One of these conditions is fibromyalgia. It is amazing people pay money for someone to use a Latin word to describe their symptom. <u>Algia</u> means pain, <u>my</u> refers to muscles and <u>fibro</u> refers to the English word fiber. This means a person is experiencing pain in the muscles. The patient knows this but using a name to describe their symptom does not teach them how to improve their health.

Let's look at other examples of what happens to people's bodies when their adrenals are not functioning properly. When a person's blood sugar starts to drop the cortisol in our system will change certain protein and fats into available blood sugar to make up for this drop. If there is an inadequate supply of cortisol then the adrenals are told to produce more and if they are too weak to do so then the blood sugar remains low. This begins the downward spiral of developing the inability to stabilize our sugar in the body. This will be discussed further when we get into the pancreas.

There are so many ladies who crave chocolate before their cycle starts. This happens because chocolate is high in magnesium. The adrenals produce progesterone to help balance her reproductive system but it takes magnesium to manufacture progesterone. Protocol dictates that she receives hormone replacement therapy which usually makes her feel better but it has nothing to do with why her body cannot produce her own hormones. Most people do not want to be responsible for their own health so in this situation she takes the hormone replacements to feel better, but her body will still be low in magnesium. You see, craving the chocolate is her friend because it is warning her that something is wrong or missing. Her health care provider is not her friend if he/she does not find out that her magnesium levels are low because there are more serious problems ahead should these levels remain low. Here is a perfect example of illustrating how we are a three-part person. Having fear in us weakens our adrenals which make so many of our hormones but we also have to have the proper nutrients to make them also.

There are people who have been slightly scratched and they look like they have been in a fight with a cat. Cortisol in the system is also an anti-inflammatory agent and if the person would have had enough cortisol this symptom would never have developed. We have just discussed a few of the symptoms that appear when the adrenals are not properly functioning and there are many more.

I stated earlier I had no intention of making this a health book because there are so many on the market today that can help you. My sole purpose is to show how we are three-part person; that said, I would like to share one more facet of chemistry in relationship to the adrenals. The adrenals need a proper balance between their sodium and potassium levels to function properly. In most of our degenerative diseases the patient is suffering from low sodium to potassium ratio. It is a fallacy to think you have to have such low sodium levels in the body. Do we not live in a sodium sack for nine months? If a person has a low sodium to potassium ratio it tells us that they are in a chronic state of unresolved stress. This stress will cause more havoc in the body than a junk food diet. Manganese is the mineral necessary to burn glucose within the cell and this mineral is also needed to elevate a person's sodium level. Again, if the sodium level gets too low compared to that of potassium, then our adrenals cannot function properly.

The adrenals producing the cortisol to elevate our sugar in times of stress is a defense system function. When under stress the adrenals burn up a lot of potassium and the mineral copper aids the loss of potassium. If you take a blood test at this point potassium levels are going to show elevated, and this is a warning that the body is under adrenal exhaustion. The body is exhausted trying to maintain high levels of cortisol to fight the stress. Blood tests at this point usually indicate a higher iron level. This is because cells are rapidly breaking down, and when they do they release iron. I do not know why but iron from broken down tissue is not eliminated, so the body stores it. The iron is moved to the liver where it is stored and when the livers ability to store it reaches a saturation point then it is sent to the pancreas. This whole process developed because the body is breaking itself down to use itself up as fuel. Any iron in the pancreas will kill the cells that produce insulin. This is another cause of why people get diabetes.

One cannot avoid stress in our life but if we are not eating the proper nutrients to replace the ones lost under stress then our bodies will eventually break down. If this happens one needs manganese, sodium, copper, and potassium. These minerals will help lower the sugar levels plus help regain the hormone imbalance the stress created. So many people (especially children) are put in a situation where they are powerless to change their circumstances; however, most adults have three choices if they are in one of these situations; (1) you can change a situation, (2) you can change yourself to fit the situation, or (3) you can leave it. If you opt not to make one of these three choices then the maladies listed at the beginning of this chapter will probably be your fate.

As I said earlier we will never have divine health without total divine forgiveness and we cannot have this without Him. He came back at Pentecost to work out in our lives everything that He worked out on the cross. This cannot happen until we trust Him and we cannot trust Him if we are still afraid of Him. He cannot take us any further into deeper spiritual growth until the fear is dealt with. For all of you who have had or are experiencing any of the problems explained in this chapter we hope we have given you a clearer understanding as to why they exist. When we totally trust Him, fear will go, AND PERFECT LOVE CASTS OUT FEAR!

People want to love and be loved, develop personal relationships, have healthy vibrant bodies, but hard as they try they never attain what they want or need because fear blocks love from coming in and the net result being the spark of life is greatly diminished. The spark is drowned out by all the energy expended maintaining the walls of protection around us. Another way to explain this process is when love is thwarted by some emotional pain we tense muscles in order not to feel the emotion and later on when we want to express love then that energy (love) is met with tension in our bodies. This tension puts further pressure on the adrenals to produce more anti-inflammatory hormones. It seemingly is an endless cycle and it cannot be broken until we deal with the root cause, and that is fear.

Please go back and reread the four versus listed at the bottom of paragraph 8 in this chapter. If God's children had these verses ground in their nature, then the root cause of fear would be removed from their lives. Notice I did not say that if they knew these verses, or memorized them, but if they had them ground into their nature. Once fear is dealt with then we are in a position to progress further into Him. This unfolds in the upcoming chapters.

If you look like the mother in the picture you may want to read this chapter again. When a person is tired in the morning, after sleeping all night, it is a good indication their adrenals are tired.

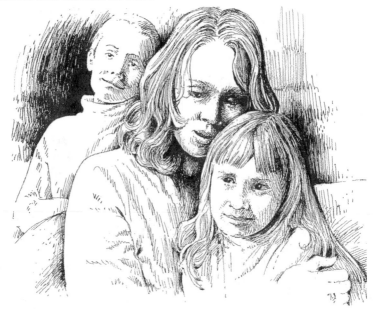

21

CHAPTER 5
THE LAVER CORRELATES
TO THE PANCREAS

The Laver is covered in John chapter 13 and this correlates to our pancreas.

The pancreas is involved in stabilizing our body's blood sugar levels and is highly involved in digestion through the production of digestive juices and enzymes. When the pancreas begins to weaken one may experience hypoglycemia, anxiety, increased sweating and mental disorientation, being more tired, getting thirstier, and experience more frequent urination. When the pancreas weakens further, one may experience loss of memory, circulatory problems and weight changes.

Let's look at the pancreas spiritually. In the Tabernacle, after the animal was slain, both the priests and the sacrifices were washed in the Laver (washbasin). Both the inside and outside of the animal was washed speaking of an outer and inner cleansing of us. I mentioned in the previous chapter that we could not trust Him until all fear is removed from our life. Once we totally trust Him then we are 100% secure in the fact that everything and everyone who comes into our life is from His hand. Regardless of how negative or painful a situation arises in our life we will know for sure He put it there to develop our character and change our nature. Nothing or no one can take this away from us. This is the root cause of jealousy: fear of losing someone or something. JEALOUSY DESTROYS THE PANCREAS!

If I say to you, "I love you, but if you love anyone else besides me, I will make your life miserable" the relationship is not on solid ground. The last part of that sentence may never be spoken but flare-ups certainly imply it. Jealousy is mean because if someone forces you to quit loving other people, regardless of gender, then life begins to get bitter. **If you are treated bitterly then life loses its sweetness, and sweetness is tied to sugar and the pancreas.**

Once we feel His love, and having fear dealt with, then we begin feeling OK about ourselves just the way we are. Not that we will not keep growing spiritually but our growth will progress only as we develop a deeper relationship with our Father. *Our growth will be a relationship, it will not be obtained by what we achieve or accomplish. Most Christian people still work hard to achieve or accomplish something to gain His favor, but that is living under the law.* They claim they are living under grace but in reality, they are still under the law. He came to set us free. By being set free we will begin to be able to see and eat life from a different perspective. Eating implies being able to absorb (digest) life. At this point in our growth we will have more power to change the way we think, which will affect our future.

We can never change our yesterday; however, we are in a better position to change our future.

Babies are not born jealous because it is a learned trait. If we are taught as children that people love then we will perceive them as such when we become adults. If we are taught that the world is a scary place then our experiences will be colored in our mind with that perception. Once we begin to see ourselves as He sees us (not what man has taught us), then the perception of ourselves begin to change. Life becomes so much more wonderful when we are free to anticipate our future from a positive standpoint. This does not mean we still will not have tragedy or disappointments but we will be free to walk through them knowing those experiences are to further develop our character and nature. Remember: jealousy hurts the pancreas! Let's discuss a few situations that develop in the body when the pancreas is not operating properly.

If you learn how to cure your own diabetes then you will have learned how to make great inroads in curing cancer because there is a common denominator in the two of them. To learn this common denominator, you need to understand that humans have two types of metabolism: one requires oxygen and one does not. We utilize both of these, depending on what is being digested: proteins, fats, or carbohydrates. Oxidative metabolism requires oxygen and we use this when were breaking down proteins and fats. Anaerobic metabolism occurs without oxygen. Anaerobic metabolism is how sugar is burned in us. Cancer cells and candida (yeast closely associated with diabetes) are both anaerobic. Since candida is a non-oxygen yeast organism, you do not have to concern yourself with this until your oxidative (aerobic) metabolism becomes weakened. For those who suffer with yeast (and millions do) you are using a bandage if you are trying to kill it. To cure it one must improve their aerobic metabolism.

When the aerobic metabolism becomes impaired then the body adjusts to using anaerobic metabolism. Fungus, cancer cells, and yeast are the result. People with yeast do not look at it as being their friend, but it is, because it is a warning of what is to come. It is a warning that sugar metabolism is dominating their body which is one step closer to becoming a diabetic. It is unfortunate that the health-care industry does not teach people how to interpret these signs or warnings. Aerobic metabolism usually declines with age and this is why cancer more often than not is associated with aging.

There are several diseases associated with declining aerobic metabolism. Even though the various diseases are given different names the root cause is the same. Digestion is so important because if our food is not totally broken down then it goes into the colon in a solution that usually becomes harder to eliminate. When we do not eliminate properly then we become toxic and the toxicity is then reabsorbed into the body. If in a toxic situation the pancreas will be over worked and consequently will be further weakened. It now becomes even harder to produce adequate insulin in the pancreas.

Insulin is the transport system for nutrients to get inside of the cells from our bloodstream; therefore, with lower insulin levels the body gets more tired. When this situation develops the body must then go into a backup system for energy. The body can take any muscle and break it down and convert 50% of it into sugar (fuel). This is the process that develops which causes so many people to waste away in many of the degenerative diseases. It is unfortunate that simple little warnings like yellow toenails, dry scalp, dry mouth or dry skin are not being taught as symptoms. If not dealt with then it will lead to further complications. What is happening is the body is flushing out its liquids trying to eliminate excess sugar. All this is going on and the end result is diabetes.

As long as people are taught that diabetes is the disease and not the symptom of something else, they are not likely to look for ways to help themselves. It is wonderful that people have insulin available to them from the doctor should the above develop in their life; however, if all they do is take the insulin then the true cause mentioned above will continue. There is more chemistry involved in the health of the pancreas than what I have mentioned; however, if the above information is not enough to stir up interest within you to search out more, then anything else I would offer would not either. It was Einstein who said, "Never regard study as a duty but an enviable opportunity to learn to know the liberating influence of beauty in the realm of the spirit for your own personal joy and to the profit of the community to which your later works belong."

I mentioned earlier I had no intention of making this a dietary book because my main focus is to point out how the various emotions tear down different parts of the body. There are many good doctors who have educated themselves to be able to help you and it would be in your best interest to find one. Years ago when I had my cancer there were two doctors who told me that my disease had nothing to do with anything I ever ate. You should know that anyone who thinks like this (even if they are a doctor) does not have their head twisted on straight. If I had believed them I would not be here today. Our libraries and the Internet are full of information to help those who are seeking the truth.

We must look at our conditions from a spiritual point of view first and then from an emotional one second. Jealousy is a derivative of fear and until fear is dealt with any attempt to try and get rid of jealousy is in vain. This is why He had to deal with our fear (the altar experience) to put us in a position to develop His character in us. Having dealt with our fear He then could deal with our jealousy. When He has removed jealousy from our nature then He has put us in a position whereby we now can develop deep personal relationships.

As we pointed out at the end of Chapter two there are seven character changes produced in us as we grow in Him. At the door experience we develop faith that gives us stability in our life. At the altar experience we begin to have virtue developed in our nature, and the laver experience gives us more knowledge. For us to develop deeper personal relationships then self-control must be made part of our nature.

CHAPTER 6
THE CANDLESTICK CORRELATES
TO THE THYMUS

The Candlestick is covered in John chapter 14, which correlates to our thymus gland.   A Candlestick (Rev 1:20 tells us the Candlestick is symbolized by the Church) with the oil (Holy Spirit) gives off plenty of light. A church without the oil has the form of godliness but lacks the power of the Holy Spirit. We will see in the few minutes how this affects our body.

The Candlestick was also called the Lampstand. Upon leaving the outer court via a veil you entered into the Holy Room. The first thing you saw was the Candlestick and the priests trimmed the candles daily. Olive oil was put on the wicks to be burned to provide light in the Holy Room. This typifies today that the Holy Spirit is to be the only light in our life. The Outer Court had no roof over it, which meant the natural sunlight was there. This typifies how Christian people today allow all the cares of this world to affect their lives. Once we learn the freedom of being able to live without some of the darkness in our nature, which He is removing, then we will want to search for more freedom.

I mentioned at the end of the last chapter that we will have learned knowledge, and the knowledge is we know He is the one who gave us our freedom; consequently, we will not let the cares of this world interfere with our relationship with Him anymore. My grandma told me when I was younger that rarely does one become a mature adult until they reach 40. She told me the reason was because when one is younger they are searching out so many interests. We experienced different things or pursued different avenues only to learn they really did not hold our interest; therefore, we walked away from them. She told me that when you are younger you are selecting a mate, developing a career and starting a family, etc. and you do not really know what interests you the most. She continued saying that when you limit yourself to about six things that hold your interest then you will be in a position to really mature. When I got to be about 37 or 38 years old I could see what she had told me, because by then I had only four things in life that I spent any time on. If this ever happens to you, you will have learned the experience of not allowing anything in this world to detract from your relationship with Him. This then puts you in a position to do develop deeper relationships. This takes us to our thymus gland.

The thymus gland lays closest to our heart and is referred to as our love gland. It stimulates the production of lymphocytes and antibodies and this gland normally decreases in size later in life. It is involved in sexual development and also helps us become more resistant to infection. When it begins to weaken one may produce too much phlegm and when it gets further weakened our resistance is lowered and then one becomes more prone to allergies and our bodies become weaker. One of its functions is to govern our heart and our circulation in the body. Until recently the consensus in the medical establishment was that this gland had little value after puberty. Their belief system was substantiated by the fact that during the Korean and Vietnam Wars, upon opening up slain victims on both sides, they found this gland had shrunk to nothing. It is true this gland shrinks when one becomes sick or dies, but when you are in love, whether you are young or older, this gland is pumped up. This is why couples getting or have just gotten married hardly ever get sick because this gland is the healthiest when we are in love.

This gland's responsibility in regard to the immune system (or defense system) is to look for anything foreign in the body and distinguish it as an enemy then it immediately begins action to destroy it. This could be a cancer cell, fungus, virus, bacterial infection, poison, a cut someplace, or something in the bloodstream not accepted as normal. Along with the thymus, our liver, spleen, lymph nodes, tonsils, appendix, adenoids, bone marrow, and small intestine make up our defense system. The thymus inter-plays with all of these. Anything foreign in the body is going to be attacked by this gland and its army. This is why before a transplant this gland must be shut down by radiation or drug treatment, and that is why such a high number of these patients are more susceptible to cancer later.

This gland is extremely damaged by stress. The stress may be in the form of being exhausted, diseased, exposure to continual noise, family problems, financial problems, job-related, and so on. If the stress is sustained for several days then the thymus shrinks to about a third its normal size. Should the body begin developing a cancer or tumor then the thymus begins working overtime to attack it. When this gland goes into an attack mode, at the same time it is stressed out, it must let secondary problems temporarily go. This could be a fungus, or maybe weaker inflamed muscles or whatever. This gland chooses to attack the most threatening problems first and will live with the secondary conditions for now hoping they can be eliminated later.

If we want to understand how this gland is to be healed we must go back to the beginning and understand how God intended and instructed our relationships and marriages to be. If marriages were bonded by His spiritual laws, then the lives of the children would have the same foundation; consequently, we would not have all the instability in our society. Notice I said His spiritual laws, not biblical laws. Most Christian people do not have His nature so the only thing they can administer is the letter of the law. Husbands use the letter of the law against their wives and husbands and wives use the letter against their children. When firm discipline is not administered with love behind the law then bitterness and resistance will result.

There are several types of love and we must understand them before we can see how each one affects the thymus gland. Look at II Peter 1:13-15! (15) Peter is talking about his death in the realm of the physical body, and in verse (14) Jesus had showed him he was going to die. Peter knew he would not enter immortality in his physical body. Why did Peter fall short? To understand where Peter went wrong we need to understand love in the Bible. There are four Greek words used for one English word love, and this is why there is so much misunderstanding concerning what the Bible says about love.

(1) Eros-sexual love, we find this mostly in Proverbs and the Song of Solomon.

(2) Storgos - Family love.

(3) Phileo - Means responsive love; I will love you if you love me, or you can count on me if I can count on you. This is the way wives are to love their husbands (we will cover this later), parents loving their children, love toward others, love of money, etc. Most marriages are consummated by eros/love, and then nourished by phileo/love.

(4) Agape - Godly love! Agape love is not human or natural. No one can have Agape love unless God gives it to them. Galatians 5:22-23 is Agape love. 1Cor 13 is Agape love. The sooner we grasp the four kinds of love and can apply them in our relationships (marriages) the sooner our thymus gland can heal. To help us understand this better let us look at why Peter knew he would die in his physical body. Jesus gave Peter the chance but Peter missed it. We cannot understand what Jesus offered Peter (and He is offering it today to us) because the Bible translators used the English word love and there is no way we could truly know what He was saying.

John 21:15-19

(15) Jesus asked Peter, lovest (Agape) me more than these? Peter replied,"Yes Lord, you know that I love (Phileo) you." You see, Jesus used the word Agape but Peter responded with Phileo. Going from the Greek to the English this comparison was completely lost.
(16) Jesus again used the word Agape and Peter responded with Phileo.
(17) the third time Jesus asked He used the word Phileo instead of Agape and this is what grieved Peter – because he then realized what had transpired. Peter said he could Phileo love Jesus, but Peter could not Agape love Him. As a result Jesus said that Peter could not overcome the last enemy, death, because he had not become an Agape lover.

The idea of being an Agape lover and overcoming the last enemy, death, centered on John, not Peter. Peter knew the difference because he was given the keys to the kingdom (2 Peter: 5-7). The last word in verse seven is love (Agape). Peter understood it, but he never attained it. It is the same principle when God took Moses to the top of the mountain and showed him the Promised Land; you see, Moses got to see it but he did not get to enter. It is the same principle for us today, because we may see or understand these principles outlined here, but if they are not in-worked into our nature then we will miss the blessings (having abundant life).

Let's bring the different aspects of love down to a more local level (in our families). Col 3:19 tells us that husbands are to love (Agape) their wines. Eph 5:25-33 the word love was translated from the word Agape: (vs. 33) 1. Agape never wants or expects anything in return. A man's love for his wife should be sacrificial, never exercising tyranny or control, but will make any sacrifice for her good. 2. A love that puts a person down isn't love at all. Any love that uses coercion instead of refining the character, which weakens the moral fiber, is not real love. Real love is the great purifier of life. 3. It must be a caring love - real love does not wish to extract services, nor tries to insure its own physical comfort is attended to; it cherishes the one it loves. 4. It is an unbreakable love, one that a man would no more think of separating from her than tearing his own body apart. Verse 33 (KJV) concludes saying that wives should fear their husbands. No wife would fear her husband who Agape loved her. The true meaning of fear biblically is awe. All wives will be in awe of their husbands if they are an Agape lover.

Anyone with common sense knows there is a great difference between men and women beyond their gender differences. For whatever reason, men think and then they feel, whereas women feel and then they think. Another difference is that men see and then they hear, whereas women hear and then they see. Neither one is the better; that's just the way we were created. With this understanding let us go back to Ephesians 5:26. Christ cleanses His church with his words; likewise, husbands are to cleanse their wives with their own words. Why? Verse 27 says Christ wants his church without a spot or wrinkle. Keep in mind that women hear first and men are to wash them with their words. This means if the husband does not use words of encouragement to her, or use words that show how much she is appreciated or enough loving words to let her know how much she is loved, then more often than not she will become contaminated with "spot and wrinkle." Verse 22 says wives are to submit to their husbands and most men love this one.

It is a God-given responsibility for man to provide for and protect his family, and in verse 28 it says we are to love our wives as our own bodies. Most men have an image of being home watching a John Wayne movie and someone crashes through the door and is a threat to them, whereupon the husband picks up a ball bat and puts an imprint on the guy's skull. For some men they are showing their obedience to verse 28; however, Christ reminds us that this act does not comply with verse 26. It is fine to protect her but if we do not apply the principle in verse 26 then we will never have a deep relationship with her. A good illustration of this principle is when a couple is getting ready to go someplace. The husband is in the living room reading the paper, ready to go, and waiting on his wife who is in the bathroom. She is getting ready and it is important to her to have his approval of how she looks (remember: it is more important for females to hear), and when she comes out of the bathroom and asks how she looks and he does not even lower the paper but just mumbles "oh fine"; he definitely did not wash her with his words. Most Christian men do not realize the biblical principle here, but whether he understands it or not and does not use the principle, his wife usually ends up becoming a nag.

Above all else men need to be respected and women need to be cherished. If he does not wash her with his loving words then she cannot feel cherished, and when she begins to nag, then he does not feel respected. It is a cycle that cannot be broken until principles He gave us are adhered too. No matter what else we may do for them and do not comply with vs. 26, then we can forget it. In Titus 2:4 the word love was translated from Phileo. Husbands are to Agape love their wives but wives are to Phileo love their husbands. In every scripture in reference to wives loving their husbands, it is always Phileo. Women are to Agape love all other members of the body, but her husband (and children if there are any) is the only one she is to Phileo love.

Remember that Phileo love expects a response and women need to hear. Wives who are not cleansed with loving words from their husbands will innately put more pressure on themselves to accomplish something else for his approval. If this then does not give her recognition for what she does or who she is, then she will start withdrawing, and one or more of her glands will become affected. Remember that the pressure she puts on herself to please him will put strain on her adrenals, and when the adrenals get tired her thyroid will have to work harder. Eventually when the thyroid gets weaker she will then start putting on weight and not too many things will put more pressure on her than this. As this process develops the closeness that they had becomes harder to maintain.

An area men need to understand is that women are many faceted and men usually are not. Men will never be but they sure would help their wives more if they understood it better. Women listen for the stove, the dryer, noise the kids are making (or not making) and all this while doing the ironing or dusting, etc. I get a kick out of a couple sitting in front of me while the kids are playing in the waiting room and she will say to him "Did you hear that?" He then replies "Hear what?" This is another way men and women are different.

Women have to learn to go against an inborn trait for them to be able to *smell the roses* that life gives us. An example of this is when a woman is driving home she is planning her evening meal, thinking about the clothes to wash, thinking about one of the children needing to go to a practice and what time another one has piano lessons. These events are played over and over in her mind. As she pulls up to a stop sign and as she is sitting there she notices a little boy in the yard playing with his puppy. She sees the little guy with her eyes but she cannot see him with her heart because she is somewhere else. Her body is in the car but she is home doing all the tasks she has played over and over. Few people live in their bodies and women especially have to work on this. If they do not, then when they get home they are already tired because they have prepared supper several times, done the laundry, etc. *God puts roses in our lives to give us a break from the pressures of life but most people are not free to smell them.*

Even though men are not many faceted, if their hearts are right, they can see their wives are over-loaded and need help with the family. I know the husband is to be the head of the household, but I totally agree with Albert Schweitzer when he said, "I do not know what your destiny will be, but one thing I know; the only ones among you who will be really happy are those who have sought and found how to serve." **You can easily tell how tall and straight a man has grown. It is seen by how flexible his heart is, which is what enables him to bend to serve.** Those men who do not are the ones who get angry when their wife is not responsive to them later at night. We cannot have a vibrant marriage if we are self-oriented. Women have to be cautious if they think they are going to make their husbands many faceted. They are setting themselves up for disappointment because it is not going to happen. Women have had more responsibility for the children in the past, still do and always will have. To try and go against the natural will only compound a mother's problems. Until men become agape lovers, the women will resent their husbands because of the extra workload they endure.

When the closeness in the relationship begins to dwindle then the principles in 1 Corinthians 13 (the love Chapter), become less of a reality in each of their lives. It was and is our Heavenly Father's intent for this type of love to be in our marriages. This is why it is so important to have instilled in our nature the attributes given to us that we learn as He walked us through the steps of the Tabernacle. At each level of progression He is stripping part of the nature that Adam gave us, which makes us less self- centered and puts us in a position to become more other-oriented. It is impossible to have a loving relationship in a marriage when either party or both are selfish.

If the only thing you want from your mate is to be together and they want the same thing, then it is impossible to fight if you get to be together. The problems begin when one wants what they want, when they want it and the other one does not or cannot comply. This is where a compromise must be worked out or a fight will begin. If the marriage is in a constant compromise state then ultimately the relationship will begin to cool down. This is the main reason God told the Hebrew people when a couple got married the man was to have no civic responsibility or go to war for one year. He was to stay home and get to know her. Everyone has had hurts and pains and the couple were to take this time to have old wounds healed so they could grow close together. This cannot happen when either or both are self-centered which means one is controlled by their five senses. God is in the process of providing in us a higher spiritual power so when situations arise in our relationship we do not respond in a manner that is painful to our mates. We were told in 1 Corinthians 13 that love is not self-seeking, rude and always protects and trusts. So basically if I truly love my wife, then it is my desire to provide an environment (wherever she is or we are) where she is free to grow and express herself to the world. If she has been thwarted, crushed, ridiculed, taught shame, etc., then she withdraws and what her true identity is (the image of God) is not what is shown to the world. It is our Heavenly Father's desire for each of us to have His image within us shown to the outside world. *When we truly love we truly have attained life, and life eagerly asserts freedoms.*

If and when both mates go through healing processes (having old hurts and wounds healed) then these traits will not be passed on to their children. Remember, the first step of forgiveness is being thankful for whatever was done to us, by whomever, and this is easily done once we realize that whatever it was has helped or strengthened us. If we do not or will not forgive them, then every time someone taps into that unresolved conflict we will respond in a manner that will hurt someone. We merely fly off the handle because someone is used as a reminder of those old past relationships or experiences that were never resolved. We may show or express a negative emotion to our mate, but in reality the true cause of our emotion is the one who wounded us and we merely direct it to our spouse.

These reactions become the teacher to our children. This then will upset the parents as they see the same traits in their children, which usually upsets the marital relationship further. As the relationship becomes more strained then more stress is put on the body. In this case it is the thymus gland that gets burdened because this is our love gland, and as mentioned earlier we become more prone to sickness when this gland is not optimal. Any time there is anything unresolved in us (the spirit man) then we begin focusing on the person who wounded us emotionally. Everything shows up in our body eventually because you begin to look like what you have been looking at over a period of time. If you are looking at someone every day that is sweet, kind, soft, considerate, loving (unfortunately not everyone gets to look at this like my wife), then your face will begin to take on the same facial features. The same holds true for negative characteristics. If we focus emotionally on people who have hurt us this then is the reason more often than not, we become like them. The more we focus on what they did to us, the more we take on the same attitudes in our own personality. When someone points this out to us we usually end up becoming angry.

It is amazing that people pray the Lord's Prayer and in one petition of the prayer we ask Him to forgive us as we forgive others. So when we will not forgive others, then we are actually asking our Father not to forgive us. *This definitely is not a good choice. The whole process keeps us burning up emotional energy to maintain our resentments and grudges.* Why do we continue to allow people, who have hurt us, to control us? If we are going to let someone control us it should be someone who is kind and sweet. If not, we make ourselves slaves to those who have hurt us. Let me repeat: we must be thankful for what was done to us because when we begin to see suffering is one of the means God uses to free us from our bondages (freeing us from ourselves), we then begin to see He is making us free to love.

It is a powerful thing to be set free because it has a tremendous effect on our health. Let's discuss for a minute what true freedom really means. Eph 5:22 states women are to be submissive to their husbands. Husbands in this verse is plural and this does not imply that she is to marry two different men. It means she is to have two husbands; Christ Jesus is her first one and her earthly husband is her second one. The wife is to be a servant to her husband in the same way Paul says he was a slave of Jesus Christ (Rom 1:1). The word slave in this verse should have been translated bond-slave (Gr # 1401).

Let us discuss the effects on our life if we were never set free. As we said earlier, our unresolved conflicts will eventually show up in our children. As this unfolds we will see how this affects our health, as well as the children. If the two parties in the marriage do not have a bonded relationship (one that develops as they are becoming one mind) then the battle lines get drawn.

Here is another way that men and women were created different. We both have a left brain and a right brain. Our left brain is our intellectual or sense of reasoning side; whereas, our right brain is where our creativity and imagination are. When we are in our left side we should be studying math and the sciences, and in our right brain, the social studies, arts, and music, etc. The man was created to be the head of the household and his wife was created to be his help meet. He should have the deepest respect for her; consequently, will ask her opinion on decisions that need to be made. Here is the real value in this: men go in their left brain at 6am., at 12 noon they go in the right brain, again at 6 pm. they go back into their left brain, and at midnight they go back to their right brain. Women are just the opposite; whatever side of the brain the man is in, the woman is in the opposite. If a married couple both get up at 6 am. and go to bed at midnight then the man is in his left brain two thirds of his waking hours, and the woman is in her right brain two thirds of her waking hours. Whenever a decision has to be made the man can only perceive it 180°; however, his wife can give him her perspective from the other 180°. This way the man is given information from both sides of the brain (part his and part hers), which gives him a 360-degree perspective. The man has now put himself in a better position to make sounder decisions.

Our society tries to convince us two males or two females can raise a child equally as well as a man and a woman. Everything else being equal this is totally impossible. If both parents have gone through healing and each is very confident and comfortable with themselves in the relationship, then the children are usually fairly balanced. When they have not the following usually develops.

If either or both parents feel insecure about themselves they will put pressure on themselves to bring up their children to be successful people, so as parents they will have proof of their worth. Since the parents have pressure on themselves, they will pass the pressure onto their children. When the mother thinks her little one should be potty trained, she will pressure the little one so mother can tell her family and friends how remarkable her little one is. There are mothers that did not want the child and the child knows it. The child will resent his mother but he/she is helpless to do anything about it because a baby is totally dependent on their parents for survival. At this point the mother is in control, and if the mother decides to leave the baby in a dirty diaper the baby may scream, but nonetheless, they will still be helpless unless someone helps them.

The story begins to change when parents want the child to start potty training. The child for the first time has some control in his life. How many toddlers have been put on the potty chair and have been told they could not get up until they go. Sometimes parents leave them sit there for an hour, with nothing happening, so the parents get them off, put their diaper on and immediately the little one fills it. The child knows exactly what he/she is doing. In the development of the child this is referred to as being anal- retentive. If parents know these warning signals they can then look within themselves for any negative motives they have applied in their dealings with the baby. If parents cannot see these warnings and correct them, the child will have more struggles in life.

How a baby is treated will determine their emotional development all the way through. Before a baby is one year-old they will have learned to trust or mistrust. The more energy a child exerts bottling up negative behavioral traits (not learned at the previous stage of development) leaves the child with that much less energy to learn what he/she is supposed to be learning at this stage. The struggles (without being corrected) will go with the child for the rest of his life. Before they are three they will have developed self-assertion and some basic independence or they will have learned shame and doubt. Before they are five they will regularly participate with others and love to explore or they will know guilt. Before they become teenagers they will know how to confidently do jobs or will have developed inferiority. Before they are 20 years old, they will pretty much be independent or be constantly in a state of confusion as to who they are. Before they get to be to 25 years old they will either be capable of developing good personal relationships or they will become more isolated in life. All through their remaining working years they will either lead meaningful lives or they will stagnate. Basically, for their remaining working years and beyond, they will feel they have contributed to society or they will live in despair.

Any time during the development of the child, whether the parents see any hidden motives or not, the parents will stand firm if they deem the Childs behavior is unacceptable. Remember: some parents must be right at all cost to prove their worth which means they will justify their position. A gap develops between the parent and the child, but down deep the child has developed a wounded spirit. The parents not understanding this start comparing the child's life to their own, showing the child has had an easier life. The child (remember he/she is now wounded) acts ungrateful and starts withdrawal of affection. Out of frustration the parents begin nagging the child, which just makes the child more stubborn and then the child starts rejecting their parent's authority. The parents getting more frustrated will put restrictions on the child to show the child who is in control and then the child becomes more rebellious. The parents begin condemning the child and defend their stand. Then the child feels everything and everyone is wrong and against them. So he/she begins doing things they were taught were wrong (this is done to punish the parents), but this only develops guilt in the child. Remember: once the mold has been set (having a painful little boy or little girl inside), no human can change this. About the only thing parents can do at this point is to ask God to purify them. Only God within can undo what man has done.

It is a miracle regardless of what station in life we are, our Father is able and willing to start immediately giving us a new view of life and begin developing it in us. When this happens our thymus gland will heal faster. We will have more meaningful relationships and we will be closer to Him. What a plan He has for each one of us if only we knew enough to reach for it. We were created to have exciting marriages where true deep love is always healing to all members in the family and each one is free to express their love. It is ours by design. Only those who yield to Him ever attain and maintain vibrant marriages. The choice is ours. Once our marriages have regained their fire then our thymus gland can heal quicker which means we will not get sick as often and we reduce the chances of getting other debilitating diseases.

Look at the miracle of this: we have more cancer, diabetes, heart problems, and arthritic conditions than ever before. Our Father has laid out a program to give us a healing. Man has spent billions of dollars on research for various diseases but our Father gives it to His children freely. This is a perfect example of why Jesus told some of them they were sighted but they were blind. Today, the answer to so many health problems is right in front of people but they are too blind to see it. This takes us to the next level.

At this point, I want to share a major roadblock that keeps people blind. It is human nature to tenaciously hold on to the system in which we were raised. We have to walk against emotional and intellectual training to make any fundamental changes in our lives. The training we were given clouds our perception of reality. There is a book written by Christopher West called "Theology of the Body Explained" that explains this wonderfully. I would highly recommend this book to anyone who is interested in knowing themselves better, and how and where they are to fit in the family.

Before we leave this chapter I would like to share one more thought. In the previous glands we discussed we attached a negative emotion to them; however, with the thymus it is not that an emotion hurts it but a lack of love will. At this stage in our development in Him we should be advanced enough that He truly is our light. When one is preoccupied or driven by fear and jealousy it is impossible to be free to love. No matter how hard one tries to love, these negative emotions constantly block us from becoming free.

An incident was just shared with us a few days ago that illustrates this point. A young father with little children was sharing the story of his childhood where his dad showed him little affection. He claimed everything was fine between him and his wife and his children; however, he knew he did not hug his children often. His wife has told him she understands why he is not affectionate. As an adult the young man has established a relationship with his dad, and that is wonderful in itself, but it does not change the fact that he is not free to be affectionate with his kids. He went on to say there is not a day in his life that he does not feel guilty because of it. His purpose for coming to see us was to tell us that he felt so jittery inside and his heart would race a lot. He went on to say that he was afraid that he was not a good dad. I might also mention that he has frequent infections.

Do you see that word afraid in reference to him being a dad? Even though it is wonderful that he loves his dad today it does not change the fact that there has been created a wall between him and his children. You see, his fear came first, and then the wall with his children came second. The wall between him and the children, coupled with his guilt because of it, makes it harder for him to keep his thymus gland healthy. For him to try to become a more affectionate father without having gone through the experiences of the altar and wash basin will only intensify the real problem. Until the real problem is dealt with we just mentioned, it is harder to keep his thymus gland healthy, and the infections will continue to be ongoing. Our Father really does have everything in the right order.

I did mention earlier that the thymus gland is near the heart and that is why it is referred to as the love gland. Proverbs 13:12 says that hope deferred makes the heart sick, but when the desire comes, it is a tree of life. This tells us that when a couple are having problems getting along, and if either one or both have no hope the marriage will get better, then this is a strain on their hearts. If and when the couple becomes closer then their hearts will become healthier. Man in his natural mind tries to convince us that cholesterol is the biggest problem with hearts. They do this to us for two reasons: (1) man in his human nature cannot heal a broken heart, which hinders him from developing a deep loving relationship, and (2) they cannot sell medicine for a heart that has healed. We will discuss cholesterol later when we get to the liver.

At this point we have a good foundation to regain our health, both physically and emotionally, but there are a few things to overcome that keep us from living life to the fullest. This takes us to the next step.

CHAPTER 7
THE SHEWBREAD CORRELATES
TO THE THYROID

The shewbread is covered in John 15, which correlates to our thyroid gland. There were 12 cakes on this table made of finely ground flour and oil. This is similar in ancient of days where the ox was tied to a grinding wheel; the ox treaded very slowly, but the grain was ground up very fine. This is very similar to what our Father does to us. He is very patient with us; consequently, He slowly, but finely, grinds His nature into us. In doing so He is in the process of removing any hidden motives or attributes in our nature that hinders our further growth in Him. This takes us to the thyroid and anger hurts this gland. We mentioned earlier that jealousy is a fear of something or someone being taken from us, whereas anger is a reaction when something or someone has taken something or someone away from us.

The thyroid straddles the windpipe and weighs about two thirds of an ounce. This gland determines the rate at which we live (do we creep slowly or race along?). It determines the rate that our cells burn fuel into energy. If it races too fast we can become jittery and nervous. The thyroid monitors cell metabolism, has an effect on our growth, our respiratory system, heart, and has an effect on our entire endocrine system. Just as a person blows into a fire to make it burn hotter, the thyroid also speeds up a person's rate of burning food into energy the same way. Stress causes our pituitary to produce a hormone to tell our thyroid to produce extra hormones. This in turn makes other things in the body go faster; for instance, this extra hormone production can cause our heart rate to elevate to a point that leaves a person exhausted. If this happens on a regular basis then the person remains thin. If our thyroid has to work extra over a period of time, because of all the extra stress, then it becomes sluggish. It then goes from a hyper to a hypo state which means there is not enough strength to blow wind on the fire to make it burn hotter; consequently, we do not burn our food up as fast and we start gaining weight. This merely adds more stress to the person and their thyroid. When the thyroid becomes hyper we are more prone to making goiters, our heart rate will increase, and we are more likely to develop tremors in our fingers, have excessive sweating, and begin losing hair. After the thyroid has been hyper it will become hypo leaving us in a state of exhaustion. When it becomes hypo we will become lethargic, we will be more prone to depression, obesity starts, and we will potentially have excessive throat soreness, lower body temperature, more prone to high blood pressure and water retention.

When we look back and see how He has walked us through the Tabernacle it becomes clear to see the changes he has made in our nature. If you were a person who had a lot of fear in you, it is now beautiful to experience life without it. The same holds true for jealousy, because if you once had it, it is remarkable to live with that weight removed from you. When these two negative emotions were removed from us we were put in a position whereby we could develop deeper relationships. If you have not experienced this yet, please be patient because the reality of being bonded to another will exceed all of your expectations.

The lack of the two negative emotions listed above will put us into a position for loving relationships; however, we still can have hidden unresolved conflicts that will test our relationships. These conflicts more often than not will express themselves in anger. I said earlier that anger is a response to something or someone who has taken something or someone from us. **When we commit everyone we know and love and all our possessions to Him, then we have removed the cause of all anger from our life.**

An example I like to use when explaining what anger is; let us suppose you are driving down the freeway in the lane you want, at the speed you want, and someone cuts in front of you and you were put into a position where you have to hit the break or jerk the car, whereupon you yell, give them a finger gesture, because they made you angry. No they did not and to illustrate this let us do it again. Driving in the same lane at the same speed, and someone cuts you off, and to your amazement you find when you look up that it is your grandma. Through your excitement you motion her off to the side of the road; you get out of your car, run up to hers and tell her how much you miss her. The first driver did exactly the same thing your grandma did but through the eyes of love, you responded different to grandma compared to him. What he did is not what made you angry but it was your response to it. You saw the first man, and what he did to you, as a thief.

Plain and simple, anger destroys us when it erupts for the wrong reason. Anger in itself is not wrong, and the reason we know this is because Christ Jesus got angry. The difference between Him and us is He never got angry against any injustices against Himself. His anger was shown when there were injustices against others. There are legitimate reasons for getting angry; for instance, we have enough technology today to feed 40 billion people on this planet, and we are not presently feeding 6 billion people. You see, there is plenty here for every man's need, but not enough for every man's greed. Anger directed wisely will change things on this earth. It merely takes men with courage and grit to make things happen

When someone gets angry because someone has taken something or someone from them the anger usually is expressed in screaming, slammed doors or withdrawing and or doing nothing. The key is when you are done expressing the anger is it gone or do you still harbor some inside? If there is any anger left inside then the thyroid will be damaged. As I said earlier the thyroid controls the speed that we live, and a person with a hyper thyroid will hurt the heart. A lot of people have unhealthy hearts because of held anger within.

Additional symptoms of hypothyroidism: one may begin experiencing dryer skin, becoming lethargic, may develop edema, cold skin, heart enlargement, impaired memory, constipation, hair loss, labored breathing, loss of appetite, heart palpitations, poor vision, emotional instability, choking easier, brittle nails, depression, muscle weakness, joint pain, and heat intolerance. In addition, ladies breast may begin to get flabby (now, how many ladies would like to get rid of anger?). Any time these emotions are a part of our nature we pay a heavy price.

I am sharing this information with you so you may have a better quality of life but there is a downside to this information if you choose not to apply it. For instance, in this case, any lady who in the future looks at her flabby breast will be reminded of the one she harbors anger against. If she does not deal with it, her anger will only be intensified, because I cannot imagine any lady voting to have flabby breast. It is amazing how our enemies control us! It seems that if we are going to let anyone control us it should be someone who is sweet, kind, considerate, etc. In the real world this is not the way it happens. Listed below are some personality characteristics that may indicate hidden anger:

1. Procrastination in the completion of imposed tasks.
2. Perpetual or habitual lateness.
3. Liking sarcastic or ironic humor.
4. Sarcasm, cynicism or flippancy in conversation.
5. Over politeness, constant cheerfulness, having an attitude of grin and bear it.
6. Frequent sighing.
7. Smiling while hurting.
8. Over controlled monotone speaking voice.
9. Frequent disturbing or frightening dreams.
10. Difficulty in getting to sleep or sleeping through the night.
11. Boredom, apathy, loss of interest in things you are usually enthusiastic about.
12. Getting tired more easily than usual.
13. Excessive irritability over trivial things.
14. Getting drowsy at inappropriate times.
15. Sleeping more than usual, sometimes 12 to 14 hours a day.
16. Waking up tired rather than rested and refreshed.
17. Clenched jaws: especially while sleeping.
18. Facial ticks, spastic foot movements, habitual fist clenching and similar repeated physical acts done unintentionally or unaware.
19. Grinding your teeth: especially while sleeping.
20. Chronically stiff or sore neck.
21. Being depressed.
22. Stomach ulcers.

Notice that I stated these personality traits may indicate hidden anger; however, there are other factors besides anger that can be a cause of the above. This is why it is so important to look at the person and not just the body. The list above deals with our emotions and mental state but we must always look at the physical body (our body chemistry) if we truly want to understand or know ourselves. A case in point: having trouble getting a good nights rest may be because of a lack of B6, or experiencing bowel problems, or having a lack of L-tryptophan, or having high blood pressure, eating too much salt, and others. The list also includes getting more tired but you can be tired from having low potassium or your iron is low, or your adrenals are exhausted, having low blood pressure, being low in zinc, being low in the B-vitamins, being low in several of the amino acids, being low in serotonin, experiencing low blood sugar, and being low in iodine because the thyroid cannot make its hormones without it. This list is not all-inclusive but it is sufficient to point out that our vitality is dependent on many factors.

We are talking about anger here: situations and or people who irritate or annoy us. We are not talking about rage, which is anger out of control. Most Christian people are taught that anger is a sin (it is impossible not to experience anger at certain times) but if you do you should not express it. Some people have tried to control their negative feelings for so long that they become unaware of feeling them. At that point one becomes convinced they do not have any hidden anger (even though they do) but nevertheless the suppressed anger will manifest itself in some way. The list above includes some of those ways the anger is expressed. If you are experiencing several of the things listed above on a regular basis then you should start looking within for any bitterness or resentment. You see anger is our friend because it is the potential tool to look within for something that hinders us from experiencing abundant life.

One thing for sure is the anger is ours even though someone else pushed our buttons that triggered it. People will do this to us all of our life, but nevertheless, the anger is ours as well as the feelings behind it. Blaming someone else will never help you grow. **There definitely are times when it is in our best interest to hold off expressing our anger but we can never afford not owning our feelings.**

As I said earlier anger will hurt the thyroid. So if you carry anger (whether it is hidden or not) you pay the price. When you are younger the thyroid will go faster and you will be very thin but when you get older it becomes hypo and then you will start putting on weight. How many women will vote for this? The weight is our potential friend because it can become the tool for us to look for the hidden problem. If you refuse to look within, for the underlying cause of your anger then the extra weight will just add to your anger. It is unfortunate the situation or person that hurt you is now controlling you.

He came to set us free but very few find it; unfortunately, this includes most Christian people because they are looking in the wrong place. They are asking

God to remove their hardships or unbearable situations when in reality He is the one who placed them in our lives. He uses those hardships to destroy our Adam nature. Christian people are looking forward to Jesus returning so they will have a better life with Him, but He returned (at Pentecost) to work within us creating His nature within us, so we may experience abundant life. *We cannot have abundant life without Him, and as I said earlier, we will never have divine health without divine forgiveness.*

Having had subtle hidden hurts removed from our heart it becomes much easier to go to the next level, which is our pituitary gland.

If the picture below looks like you in traffic then you may want to read this chapter again.

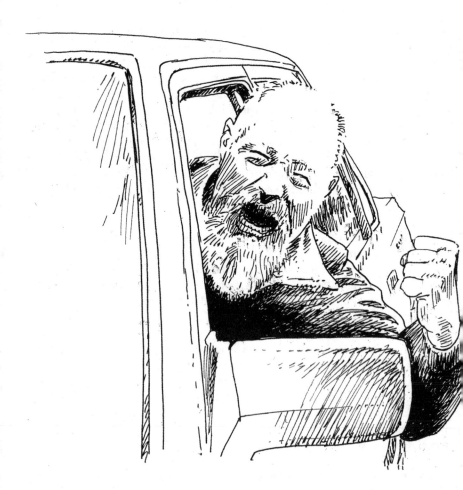

CHAPTER 8
THE GOLDEN ALTAR OF INCENSE CORRELATES TO THE PITUITARY

The golden altar of the incense is covered in John chapter 16 and it correlates to our pituitary gland. This gland is involved in human growth hormones and in the regulation of the thyroid and adrenal glands. It is also involved in our ability to break down fat. If this gland becomes less efficient you might experience more frequent urination and also have excessive thirst. A person at this point may experience glandular stimulation and when this gland becomes further weakened one may start experiencing weight on the hips and on the thighs. Another development may be you will begin having trouble losing weight anywhere and the persons glandular secretions will slow down making them slower in general. The hypothalamus (a portion of our brain) uses our five senses to gather information and then determines what our body needs to stabilize itself against the outside world. This information is sent to the pituitary gland and then the pituitary through its secretion of hormones sends signals to the other five glands below it instructing them what hormones they are to produce to keep us stable against the outside world and enabling us to maintain a healthy state.

The following is a list of hormones produced by the pituitary gland and their effects in the body: (1) growth hormone (somatotrophin)-promotes proteins synthesis, increases breakdown of fats for energy, increases bone growth, helps tissue repair, and regulates growth, (2) thyroid stimulating hormone (thyrotropin)-regulates the thyroid gland by stimulating production of thyroid hormones, (3) adrenocorticotropic hormone (acth)-stimulates adrenal cortex to produce cortisol and other stress management hormones, (4) luteninizing hormone(lh)-stimulates reproductive glands to produce estrogen and testosterone, (5) follicle stimulating hormone (fsh)-stimulates estrogen production and ovulation, (6) prolactin-stimulates development of breast tissue and the secretion of milk, (7) melanocyte stimulating hormone-stimulates melanocytes in the skin to produce melatonin for skin pigmentation, and also stimulates ones sex drive, (8) oxytocin-stimulates uterine contractions during childbirth and production of breast milk, (9) antidiuretic hormone (adh)-inhibits the formation of urine by reducing the amount of water secreted by the kidneys. For all the responsibility this gland has in keeping the other glands in the endocrine system working properly it is no wonder they call this gland the master gland.

In John 16:23-24 Jesus is teaching us a new way to pray because he was symbolically participating in the Golden altar of incense, which is an intercessory prayer altar.

As Christ Jesus leads us through the Tabernacle (the Tabernacle that we are) He exposes our inner conflicts that must be placed on the altar to be killed. Paul said, "I die daily"! Any portion of our mind (part of our soul) that does not think like the mind of Christ is our flesh. The candlestick and shewbread experiences are both an inward working of serving our needs. No one can live up to their potential if they are weighted down with jealousy, fear, anger, and the other negative emotions. He takes care of our needs as He removes those traits out of our nature. As He progressively does this within us we then become more God-centered instead of self-centered. When the altar of incense is burned in our nature then we take our prayers and praise outward for other people's needs to God, instead of our own needs.

So many preachers preach in their sermons that we are to die for Jesus. He does not want us to die for Him but to die to ourselves so we can truly live for Him. **When we are put into the position to truly live for Him then other people and their emotions no longer control us.** Here is the bottom line: the pituitary is often referred to as our master gland and control freaks continually overwork their pituitary. Control freaks are constantly manipulating others so they (the controllers) get what they want. Catastrophe happens to controllers when something develops in their life, or in the life of one of their loved ones, and the controller is helpless to do anything about it. In a business situation a boss who is a controller can get away with it because he/she controls the purse strings, but it is quite different in family situations. When a child grows up and gets married and he or she does not live by the standards of the controlling parent and the child and their mates are not confrontational people, then the manipulating game continues. You can bet the controlling parent will not change; consequently, a division in the family will develop.

I have heard a lot of older people say they have learned to keep their mouth shut because it saves a lot of trouble; however, their insides are buzzing wishing things or situations were different. No matter what course of action a controller takes, whether it is a verbal expression to control others or becoming silent and still feeling the same emotion, the end result is the same on the pituitary gland. This is one of the causes of people developing tumors. So many tumors develop because of pituitary gland hormone imbalances. Notice I said one of the causes because not all tumors are because of this. For instance, I have a friend who had a blow to his head that blocked his oxygen flow to the area and a tumor developed. This is why it is so important to look at the person and not just their body when one is sick because not everyone who gets a particular disease gets it for the same reason as someone else.

The key for a controller getting healed was illustrated for us by Paul when he said "I die daily." As I pointed out earlier the key to inner peace is coming to the realization that everything and everyone in our life is there because of our Father's hand. Control freaks are severely threatened by anything or anyone that begins to break their domain. If we learn to live for His will instead of our own (that is what Paul meant when he said "I die daily"), then what others choose to do will not upset us. We all make choices daily because of situations put in our lives and we constantly analyze that information by our computer (our brain). We are limited to the choices we make by the information in our computer and controlling people live and believe everyone should think like they do. That is impossible but controlling people have not learned this. If we have learned something that someone else has not, it is something to be grateful for but never to be proud of. If we become proud then our nature will be critical and condemning. That was Dale Carnegie's big three: criticize, condemn and complain! For a controller to try and change is an act of futility until he has had the other emotions we have discussed in previous chapters dealt with. To try not to be a controlling person when you still have fear in you will only lead to failure. This is why He progressively walks us through the tabernacle within. Each step or lesson learned is the foundation for the next step or lesson.

As He progressively burns His nature into us at each position in the tabernacle then we are in the position to learn what He wants to give us at the next higher level. By saying the next higher level I am referring to a deeper relationship with Him. Ephesians 4:15 says "but speaking the truth in love, may grow up into Him in all things which is the head, even Christ." Notice it says into Him and not unto Him! This is our Fathers purpose for his elect and that is to make them to become like His first Begotten Son. The writer of Hebrews tells us that Christ Jesus is our great High Priest and that He is our forerunner. If He is the forerunner that means He intends for us to run after Him and this takes us to the next step.

The process He is taking His elect through is for the purpose of preparing them to reign with Him. Christian people have a mistaken notion that they are going to die and reign with Him, but it simply is not going to happen. Revelation 3:21 (KJV) says "to Him that overcomes will I grant to sit with Me in My throne, even as I also overcame, and am sat down with My Father in His throne." Notice it says in My throne and not on My throne. The word in implies a position of authority with Him and not a place to set on. **When we die to Him then the root cause for needing to control (this includes ourselves), is removed from our life.** There are not too many things that can happen in a family that is more conducive to healing than having a controlling member get healed. Let's move on to the next step of character development.

CHAPTER 9
THE ARK OF THE COVENANT
CORRELATES TO THE PINEAL GLAND

The pineal gland is the bio-clock that regulates menstrual cycles. It is the psychosomatic center and it monitors fear in the body. It is often referred to as the spiritual gland and there have been experiments done on how to expand or enlarge this gland. It was thought if they could do this then that person would be more intelligent and have more power. If this gland becomes weakened then one might experience over-stimulation of their sex glands. This could possibly result in longer menstrual cycles and more mental problems. If the condition worsens then the periods start to get irregular and become shorter in duration. When this happens one could begin experiencing excessive worry and fear.

The word for Ark means chest in which something is hidden in secret. This refers to the deeper hidden purposes in God's word that are only revealed to those who seek Him. What He is revealing to those who seek Him is what He is doing to us, and for us, so that we will come into our inheritance. God had Moses place in the Ark:

1. Manna: this represents the hidden deeper meanings in God's word.

2. Aaron's rod that budded: this represents God's Manifested Sons who will grow into maturity and rule (Revelation 2:26-27). The manifestation of the Sons of God is covered in the 8th chapter of Romans. It is amazing to me that this subject (the manifestation of the Sons of God) is never preached in churches or on television or the radio. Most preachers preach what they think or expect God to do but God tells those who have eyes to see and ears to hear what He is going to do.

3. Table of stone: this is what the 10 Commandments were written on. This is symbolic of what He is doing in our life. In the Old Testament He wrote His Laws in stone but in the New Testament He is writing His laws (His nature) in our heart.

The Ark is covered in John 17. John 17:21 says, "that they all may be one, as You, Father, are in Me, and I in You; that they also may be one in us." There are times that we all feel isolated or all alone and this is when we need to read John 17. This chapter explains why we are where we are because Jesus has prayed that we may be one with the Father as He is. Do we really want God to answer that prayer or do we have some other goal for ourselves? God reveals in this chapter His purpose is not just to answer our prayers but through prayer we might come to know Him. This is a prayer God has to answer because Jesus prayed it. How can any Christian believe a prayer of Jesus will not be answered? Look at versus 21 again: "that they <u>all</u> may be one." Do you see the word all in this verse? Only if you know Him will you have eyes to see or ears to hear so that you can understand the magnitude of this verse.

You see, God does not ask us if we want to go through a difficulty, defeat or the loss of a loved one. He allows these experiences in our life for His purpose. The experiences we go through will either make us kinder and develop His character in us or they will make us more critical and harsh. If we truly can pray as He did in Matthew 26:42 ("Your will be done") then John chapter 17 is very comforting. When we line ourselves up to His will we will not become small-minded and cynical. At that point we have the assurance our Father will complete His will in our lives.

We now come to the point on how all of this affects our pineal gland. It is similar to the 10 Commandments in that if you do not break the 10th one you will not have broken the first nine. You see, it is not that a particular emotion hurts this gland as much as it is having all the other damaging emotions removed from our life (and having the corresponding glands healed we have mentioned in previous chapters) then the pineal gland will automatically be healthier. Remember, the priest went through the door of the Tabernacle and as he did his duties he kept walking further inside. This is the same pattern that Christ follows in our hearts today. At each step of the way He is healing the emotions we have been discussing. This progressive working gets easier at each step or level.

As mentioned earlier, He is stripping away a portion of our Adam nature each step of the way. As that happens at each step He puts us into a position of regaining our health and getting closer to having abundant life. Also, this gland has some control over our sex glands and our sex drive is definitely a sign of life. Everyone should have a strong sex drive because if you do not you become very lethargic. Without a sex drive you begin losing interest in life. This has nothing to do with sex but with our drive to experience life whether we are married or not. It has everything to do with our drive for life to pursue many other interests we enjoy. I pity the poor soul who only wants to come home and watch television or play computer games. The mind is such a precious gift to waste it away. I am amazed at the number of middle-aged and older people who respond by saying, "I do not know" when I ask them what is their favorite thing in life to do. What a sad thing to have to write on someone's tombstone. If we do not have a reason to jump out of bed in the morning then life is passing us by

Mankind has been trying for 2000 years to prove Him wrong. He said, "I am the life." Oh yes, people can do lively things but only He can put life in us so that we can enjoy them. Man is usually in the wrong place at the wrong time trying to accomplish good things but in the wrong way. *We will never have peace in the world by bombing or starving people. Peace will never come until He fulfills His purpose in His people.* <u>If there is righteousness in the heart there will be beauty in the character. If there is beauty in the character there will be harmony in the home. If there is harmony in the home there will be order in the nation. If there is order in the nation there will be peace in the world. Anything else is man using bandages to cover symptoms. Until God changes the nature of man the terrible conditions on this earth will continue.</u> It is impossible to be the best possible spouse, parent, neighbor or employee until God changes ones nature and that is why He walks us through the Tabernacle: to accomplish His purpose within us.

Until we begin to see all mankind as Christ sees them we will remain critical and judgmental. Christian people are Christians because they have responded to the free gift of faith He offered them. Notice that I said free gift of faith and not free gift of salvation as it is commonly preached. Please stay with me for a minute and we will see how this applies to our pineal gland. You see, He gives us faith and then salvation follows. Ephesians 2:8-10 says "for by grace are you saved through faith: and that not of yourselves; it is the gift of God: not of works, lest any man should boast. For we are His workmanship, created in Christ Jesus unto good works, which God has before ordained that we should walk in them." It has been commonly taught that this passage says that salvation is a gift of God but simple grammatical instruction shows us that this is not the case. The verse says, "and that not of yourselves; it is the gift of God." In these 10 words of scripture there are two pronouns: "that" and "it" and according to proper English point back to an antecedent noun. The noun salvation is not in this text so these two pronouns cannot refer to salvation (the word saved is used but in this verse it is a verb). The only nouns in this verse are grace and faith and since grace is an attribute of God the pronouns "that" and "it" can only refer to faith. So we can read the verse as follows: "and that faith is not of yourselves; it (faith) is the gift of God." It is so important to see it is not our faith that saved us but it was His, and then we come to the realization that He has not revealed this yet to the unsaved. It is not their (the unsaved) choice that this (His faith) has not been revealed to them yet. When we have this reality deeply embedded within us we will quit being so judgmental and critical of them and their behavior. Most Christian people somehow believe that the sins of the body are so much worse than the sins of the disposition. Let me repeat a thought I shared in chapter 3: Christians routinely skip over Matthew 7:1-2, which says, "Judge not, that you be not judged. For with what judgment you judge, you will be judged; and with the measure you use, it will be measured back to you." Whether you know and understand the magnitude of these last two versus does not change the fact that if you are critical and judgmental your pineal gland (and the other six glands in the endocrine system) will never be totally healthy.

It is imperative that we get beyond the babes in Christ mentality regarding so many misunderstandings of various versus as they are taught. To properly understand these verses from our Father's point of view makes it more conducive for us to regain our health, both mentally and physically. The entire chapter of 1Cor.15

deals with Resurrection. The common perception of this verse is that in the future graves are going to be opened up and people will be rising up out of them. To have a false perception of the Resurrection will only give you a false perception of God's redemptive work throughout the ages. 1Cor.15: 22 says, "For as in Adam all die, even so in Christ all shall be made alive." In the new Testament Concordant Literal this verse reads as follows: "As in Adam all are dying." This verse is not contrasting dead bodies and walking bodies. It is contrasting the dying process and the life process in Him. The dying process drags man into sin, sorrow, and death, whereas being " made alive" means He imparts His life into us. Both terms "are dying" and "shall be made alive" implies an action in progress.

The Resurrection is not something that is going to happen sometime in the future. Jesus rebuked Martha (John 11:22-25) for thinking this way. He told her that the Resurrection and The Life was standing right there beside her. The Resurrection was not something that happened to Jesus or an event where He was; the Resurrection was and is A MAN! To possess the Man and to enter into union with the Man is experiencing the Resurrection, for the Man is the Resurrection. Jesus was praying to the Father (John 17:21) asking that we become one with Them (He and the Father). When this prayer is answered in our life then we will have experienced the Resurrection. It is not a matter of going anywhere, but if we do not have eyes to see and ears to hear then we cannot see it (understand it). The only thing left then is to be able see it in the natural. So many of God's beautiful truths in His word have been marred by the carnal mind of men. Oh that God would remove the veil from our Adam mind so that we can see His truths regarding His purposes for our lives. If He does not, then we will remain babes in Christ, instead of maturing into Sons of God. *If we remain babes then we will always lack His Peace, and without His Peace we will lack the strength and vitality that is our birthright as His sons. This is what disease is (dis-ease)!*

Our Father gives us the natural to show us spiritual realities. By understanding the law biogenesis the above paragraph becomes very clear. Through another pen this law was beautifully explained. This law states that all life comes from pre-existing life. You cannot produce life from inorganic chemical substances. A higher life must invade a lower life to produce life in the lower life. This is how the inorganic, nonliving mineral elements of the earth are raised up into the organic kingdom of living things. Inside the seed is a germ of life and man plants this into the earth (the kingdom of the dead). If the earth has the right amount of water, air, and the right temperature, the seed germinates and the life within the seed begins to grow. The shell of the seed breaks and the life from the seed releases into the earth. As the life is released it seizes upon the chemical elements in the earth, converts them into food, and then builds up living tissue out of matter that never lived before. The inorganic chemicals become organic tissue.

The same process happens spiritually. The Holy Spirit touches with His divine life, the dead souls of men and gaps the bridge between the natural and the spiritual, and endows them with His holy and eternal divine qualities and produces within them the ability to see the kingdom of God. Ephesians 2:1-5 portrays this beautifully. It states how He has (past tense) quickened us. His indwelling life grips our heart, fills our mind, and this will begin to transform our lives. **When He changes our minds then our emotions will become more stable, which enables our bodies to be renewed as well.** Please read this last sentence again. It is common sense that we should exercise and eat right, but doing so without peace of mind is like swimming against the current. Our inheritance is abundant life but man is trying to pursue it the wrong way. *I said before and I'll say it again, if you want more than the masses have, you cannot do what they do. When the principles in the three previous paragraphs have been inworked into our nature, then our pineal gland is in a position to be healthy.*

I would like to add another thought in regards to the three previous paragraphs. 1 Tim 1:4 tells us not to "give heed to fables." 2 Tim 4:4 says, "and they will turn their ears away from the truth, and be turned aside to fables." I said before and I will say it again, if we do not know where we came from, and who we are, and why we are here, we easily become prey to fables regarding where we are going. John 14:1-7 reads as follows: "Let not your heart be troubled; you believe in God, believe also in Me. In my Father's house are many mansions; if it were not so, I would have told you. And if I go to prepare a place for you, I will come again and receive you to Myself; that where I am, there you may be also. And where I go you know, and the way you know." Thomas said to him, "Lord, we do not know where you are going, and how we can know the way?" Jesus said to him, " I am the way, the truth, and the life. No one comes to the Father except through Me. If you had known Me, you would have known My Father also; and from now on you know Him and have seen Him."

Now look at how <u>most preachers preach</u> these verses: "let not your heart be troubled; you believe in hell, believe also in heaven. In heaven there are many mansions; you know I have told you this and have described its beautiful golden streets many times. I'm going to heaven to prepare a mansion just over the hilltop for you, and if I go and prepare a mansion for you, I will come again and take you away to heaven, that where I will be you will be also. And you know well that I am going to heaven, and you know the way to heaven. And Thomas said unto him, Lord, we did not know you were going to heaven, and how can we know the way? Jesus said unto him, I am the way, the truth and the life. No man shall ever get to heaven but by Me. If you had known me, you should have known My Father also; but when you get to heaven you shall know Him and you shall see him." The subject of the 14th chapter of John is not heaven!

Jesus did not come to reveal some geographical location but to reveal our Father. Becoming One in Christ is our destination; it is not going to heaven. He tells us in these verses we are going to the Father. The word heaven does not appear once in this entire chapter. If anyone wants to count the number of times the word Father is mentioned in this chapter they can, it is 23. In this chapter Jesus used these words to help bring us into a living relationship with our Father. These verses have nothing to do with giving us a road map to some far-off galaxy.

If my Father is "in heaven" then I can expect from Him only things that come from Him and are heavenly in character, and will make me heavenly. All that comes to me from heaven will make my life and my world more heavenly. In the 10 Commandments the first one says we are to have no other God but Him, the second one says we are to have no graven images before us, and the third one says we are not to use any profanity. We cannot break the first one if we have the right picture of Him which was shown to us by His Son. We will not break the second one if we have the correct picture of Him and not the one that is commonly portrayed. The third one will not be broken if we think about the picture as He truly is. **The majority of Christians hallow God's name with their lips, but defile Him in their hearts, attitudes and actions. They read into God's nature their own ignorance and prejudices, and make Him altogether one like themselves. Very few people take the time to use their brain as long as their prejudices are alive and well. They may not make any images out of wood and stone, but they will make one out of the materials their own hearts supply; consequently, He is made out to be harsh, narrow-minded, vindictive, bigoted, and cruel as they are.** Believing in the incorrect picture does nothing positive for our physical or mental state of being.

I have mentioned several times Christian's become prey to fables. One of the main reasons for this is they start reading their bible beginning with the first book. They then listen to a preacher tell them what is coming, and what God is going to do when He decides to end the whole thing. If you do not know how things are really going to turn out, it becomes easy for someone to teach you fables. What we really should do is go to the end of the bible to see how it ends. From this viewpoint we can read the entire bible and see how each book and chapter leads to that end. Revelation ends with "I make all things new"! When we begin to see every verse with that understanding, then we can easily see any interpretation that does not line up with the way God says it is going to end, makes us prey to believing fables.

If you have any symptoms listed at the beginning of this chapter and have no interest in what we have mentioned in the last couple paragraphs then the fact remains you will have the symptoms for a long time. We will never have good health without a solid mind, and it is hard to maintain a solid state of mind without knowing who we really are and where we are going. Our Father has freely given us the answer to these two questions that have been asked since the beginning of time, if we only have the eyes to see (understand).

When we do not understand these verses in John then it becomes problematic for God's children to live in the now. They are either living in the past thinking of what He did for them at Cavalry or they are thinking about what they hope He will do for them when they die. These verses in John were recorded before He went to the cross, so the place He went to prepare for us was Calvary. At the Ascension He went to the Father (Spirit) so that He could return at Pentecost to abide in us. If you look up the word mansion in the above verses you will notice it means tabernacle. He said He wants to tabernacle in man. To those who have eyes to see know that we are the mansions He referred to in these verses. It is not some cabin out there in some gloryland. When we get our minds off fables then we are free to live in the reality that He is, which enables us to live in the now. If we do not live in the now it is impossible to have abundant life (which is what He came to give us) and anything short of this will rob us of our health and vitality. This is the bottom line!

Before we go into body chemistry I would like to discuss several other emotions that hurt the body besides those of the endocrine system. We will do this in the next chapter.

CHAPTER 10
OTHER EMOTIONS

In the previous chapters we pointed out all the negative emotions affect every part of the body but each one of them discussed had a direct hit on a specific gland in the endocrine system. There are additional emotions that specifically hit other parts of the body. The liver is hurt by **resentment**. Again, all the negative emotions hurt the liver but resentment is a direct hit. The liver supposedly performs over 1000 functions but at this point I want to mention just one of them. Cholesterol is on most minds because of a massive media blitz. Whatever your cholesterol registers in a blood test only 20% of that number comes from your diet. A person's liver accounts for most of the rest of that number. The liver takes two components of the B- complex family and makes another product called lecithin. There are no dietary rules that apply to everyone; however, for a good number of people mixing a good cold-pressed safflower oil and a good organic lecithin will do wonders for cleaning your veins and arteries. In this chapter we are still talking about emotions so I do not intend to go any further into body chemistry here.

Several years ago ABC ran a segment on 20/20 about a group of people who were all over 100 years old. There was a common denominator in all of them: (1) they all had a high degree of faith in God, (2) they all were still working, (3) they all had lost mates and most of them had lost children. One particular old man stood out regarding what we are talking about here. I may not remember all the details of the story but the bottom line is accurate in relationship to what we are sharing. He was a black man and said he could remember how he was treated. We know the slaves were freed after the Civil War but many were treated as such many years after that. If I remember right, he was 104 years old so he would have never been a legal slave but he did remember being treated as one. He said that God had been good to him because he got to see all those men dead. Hugh Downs asked the man if he was born again and the man replied that he knew he was. The man said the reason he knew he was born again, was because he had young looking hands and young looking feet because he had forgiven them all, because he knew that He lived in his heart. In my mind and in my heart his life exemplified what true divine forgiveness will do. **You see, man freed him from slavery but only Christ Jesus could free him from himself.**

This concept is a major problem in the African American community today. White men freed them, educated and helped them financially; unfortunately, there are people who have convinced them they should be paid for the bondage that their forefathers suffered. The problem is they have been manipulated into looking backward to see <u>what was</u> instead of looking at <u>what is</u> today. If I chose to, I could look backward and see they owe me because my ancestors were killed trying to free theirs. If any of us choose to look backward to see the negative, then we put ourselves in a position to harbor resentment. We cannot be free people if we choose to allow anyone else to put resentment in us. If and when we allow this to happen we definitely are in bondage quite unlike the man mentioned above. Why do we allow other people to control us?

George Washington Carver was the black man who developed so many uses from the peanut. When he lived black people had to get off the sidewalk when white people approached them. One day George and his friends were walking down the sidewalk when three white boys approach them. Before George and his friends stepped aside the white boys shoved them and George fell into the street. When he stood up he was wet and muddy. The white boys laughed as they went walking on and George's friends ask him if he was going to do anything about it. George told them no because he refused to let another person control him. George remained free to go back to his research regarding peanuts. Had he gone back to his study holding anger and resentment against those boys who did what they did to him, it would have hindered him from his studies. George would not allow this and consequently he accomplished so much in his life. What a tremendous lesson he learned that most people, whether black or white, never learn. *What a tremendous price to allow a person who has done an evil deed to us control us.* George did not know this but he put his liver in a position to continually serve him. For those people who have not learned this eventually find their liver not doing some of its functions and they end up going to a doctor and taking medications for some ailment. What an awful price for bondage.

Worry hurts the stomach. When Christ Jesus walked on this earth He told us to cast our burdens onto him. When we do not life's problems become very heavy. When we cannot trust Him for today's problems then responsibility for those problems become ours, and the weight of them overwhelms us. It is one thing to trust Him for our redemption but it is altogether different to trust Him to carry us through our daily lives. Worry is something that is learned because you did not worry the day you were born. When people ask me about what to do for worrying I always tell them that they are not the smartest person in the world nor are they the dumbest. I tell them that they are not the dumbest person in the world because they were smart enough to learn to worry. I tell them that if they are smart enough to learn how to worry then they are smart enough to learn to quit worrying. This is why having Him develop His nature in us, as He walks with us step-by-step through the Tabernacle, is so important because the foundation for worry is fear. **If and when in my development in Him He instills in my consciousness that everything comes to me through His hand, then I am secure that everything will be all right. This then leaves me with nothing to worry about ever again.**

This does not mean we will not have any cares anymore nor will we stop planning ahead but we will not worry about the outcome. He does not have the answer to our problems; He is the answer. Very few Christians get to the point that they know He is the answer. For most Christians who went to Sunday school as a child, later attended church, will find on their deathbed the only Jesus they know is the One who walked in Palestine 2000 years ago. They know him as the Savior who healed the sick, cast out demons, raised the dead, fed the multitude, but they know nothing of the Christ within working out in our lives what He worked out on the cross.

I have heard many Christians through the years say they would like to have Jesus sit down and talk to them, but it is amazing His disciples did that for 3 1/2 years and it did not help them. They watched Him do everything He did for 3 1/2 years and listened to Him for the same length of time. After all that time together Peter could still cuss like a sailor and Judas could still betray Him. It was not until after Pentecost when He moved within that they began to see the things He told and showed them when He walked with them. He could and still can do more within than He ever could do without and yet people still want to see the flesh man again. He took Himself from their eyes so He could give Himself to their hearts and if we still want to see Him with our eyes then that means we cannot see Him in the spirit. *If we cannot see Him as He is (verses as He was) then we are being robbed of our true inheritance, which is a deep personal relationship with Him.* Anything short of this will leave us trying to change our lives but it will only be external.

Each one of us has two natures inside of us and each is like a little dog. One of them is black and one of them is white. The one you feed will be the strongest and he will chase the other one from the food. The same process is going on in each of us. The more one feeds the human nature of Adam the more the Christ nature will have a hard time getting you to feed it until some day you will no longer want to feed at His table. At that point you will no longer have the desire to talk to someone about Him because you have not fed the Christ nature within you. When you feed the Adam nature it does not take much to lose your temper if someone crosses you. There are all kinds of possibilities living with and around people who constantly feed the Adam nature: there is greed, violence, dishonesty, distrust and others. We choose whether we want to worry about all of these conditions around us and if we do our quality of life is challenged.

Some people become obsessed with things (this is the root cause of envy) and when they do it hurts their spleen. When this happens it becomes harder for them to become inspired. At that point it becomes easy to fall into the trap of thinking thoughts like what difference does it make? *Some people were criticized so much as little children they grew up feeling they were always disappointing someone and would always be a failure*. These people build a box around themselves for security because if they do not venture out-of-the-box they cannot experiment with other aspects of life. They maintain such *rigid thinking* on how life should be lived that their joints become rigid also because our joints represent free movement in our body. It is so sad so many people have body ailments because of unconscious conflicts. *Only He can deal with these conflicts; unfortunately, man has spent the last 2000 years trying to prove Him wrong.*

Grief is another emotion quite unlike all the rest because it is a derivative of love. All of the other emotions come from our Adam nature. If you have lost a loved one and are grieving it is a blessing that you can, because you had the privilege of experiencing loving them. It is very healthy for us to express grief, but if we continue grieving for an extended period of time it will hurt our lungs. I met a man who lost his wife from cancer in the fall of the year. The following year in the spring he was in the hospital for chest pain. They could not find anything wrong with him so they gave him medicine and sent him home. He had eight children and the youngest ones were still home. At this point he had not gotten over losing his wife and I explained to him how grief hurts the lungs. I told him if he could have his wife back for five minutes she would tell him that life will never be the same, although it could be better. She would tell him that he was not doing justice to the children and for him to do so, he must let her go. He came back to see me in a couple weeks and his pain was all gone.

I cannot emphasize enough if we want a total healing we must look at the entire person and not just the body. So many people are dying inside because of past pain and failures and if we want to help them we must become the tool to help the little boy or the little girl inside of them. If we cannot discern this in other people what real value are we to mankind? It is sad because **loneliness** is the greatest disease in our country and hardly anyone sees it in other people. We may not all know how to build bridges or be brain surgeons but we all can sit down and hold the hand of someone lonely. It costs us nothing to do so but it takes a soft heart to be able to see it in them. When this is developed in us our lives we will be the richer for it. It was and is and always will be my intent to share what our Father has done, is doing, and will continue doing in His children to develop them into the nature of His Son.

Everything we have shared so far in the previous chapters has dealt with the emotions and their effects on our physical body; however, for us to have vibrant lives we must understand body chemistry and its effect on us. We mentioned earlier that it is not our intent to make this a health book because there are so many on the market today; however, I do feel there are some basics most people do not understand so we will discuss them in the next few chapters.

Before you go to body chemistry please look at the following diagram. You will notice the pictures in the center row and on the left are in the diagram in chapter two. On the right side we have added the corresponding personality traits that are driven into our nature as each of the emotions have been healed. By the time you have progressed to the top your mental and emotional makeup will be such you will be able to weather any storm you face. Then the only thing left for us to have vibrant health is to understand and apply proper body chemistry.

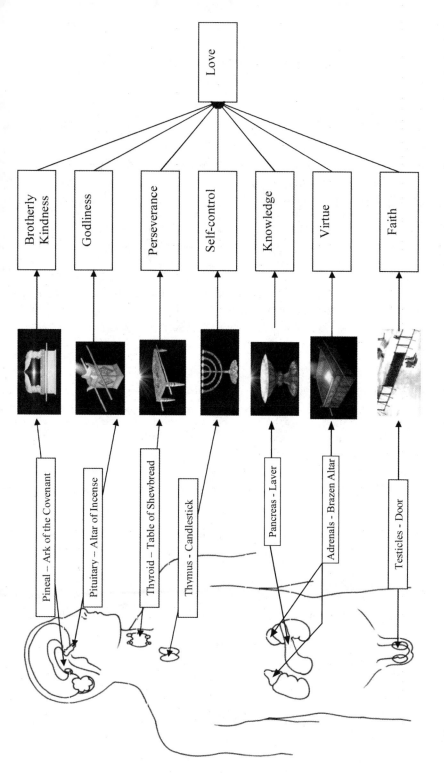

Love

Brotherly Kindness — Pineal – Ark of the Covenant

Godliness — Pituitary – Altar of Incense

Perseverance — Thyroid – Table of Shewbread

Self-control — Thymus - Candlestick

Knowledge — Pancreas - Laver

Virtue — Adrenals - Brazen Altar

Faith — Testicles - Door

CHAPTER 11
BASIC BODY CHEMISTRY

Our Father created us with body chemistry when balanced and maintained will enable us to live a long and healthy life. If we are healthy our acid/alkaline balance will be slightly alkaline. This is not hard to do, and you will want to once you understand its value. *Plain and simple: if we are too acid we are going to be sick and when a person gets totally acid they die.* All illnesses are a warning that our body chemistry is out of balance. If everyone understood this simple point, that when they get sick they merely have to ask themselves what do they need to balance their pH? If people could get out of the mindset of thinking they have some disease then they would be free to focus on what do I need to do to change my body chemistry? Understanding this frees us from the fear of what do I have? People that understand body chemistry know if they are told 10-20 years in the future they have cancer, they automatically will know all they have to do is find out what they need to change their body chemistry and they will get their healing. Ignorance is very expensive! *When you do not understand what you have or how you got it then it becomes easy for someone to scare you and talk you into something that is not in your best interest.*

When we discussed the emotions we pointed out that every negative emotion forces our body into producing more acid. On top of that what most people eat produces even more acid. The more acid buildup we have the more we will age. Food that is commercially processed is very acidic and unfortunately this is what most people live on. The agricultural industry uses so many chemicals in raising crops that the food processors have to use so much sugar in their products to kill the chemical taste.

A body that has a proper pH cannot be a home for fungus, bacteria or viruses. These all thrive in an acid body. The germ theory in connection with disease is not correct. Hospitals are the worst place to go if you do not want to get sick, and who disinfects more than hospitals? Germs and viruses are not the problem; we are! Germs and viruses live on anything that is dead and if they invade our bodies and there is nothing dead inside for them to eat, then they die. Since people do not digest or eliminate properly they then have so much dead material in them and this is sheer food for these nasty invaders. People are not being taught how to stay healthy and consequently we have a very sick society. The entire medical community is not wellness orientated it is sickness orientated. Do you realize that if everyone in this country became healthy the U.S. economy would go into a nosedive?

When we become too acidic this means we have less oxygen in our bloodstream. One of the main problems in heart disease is a shortage of oxygen. People get cancer because oxygen cannot get into the cells and the glucose within ferments. In both cases an over acidic body is the culprit.

Acidosis is a condition that develops when carbon dioxide accumulates in the tissues; consequently, they no longer can utilize oxygen. When this condition worsens then people begin having trouble breathing because basically they are suffocating.

There are two pH systems in our bodies and they need each other. The first one is in our bloodstream and it is to be alkaline slightly and the other is in the stomach and it is to be acidic. Man's understanding is always backwards and this is especially true in understanding digestion. When the body has a symptom of acid indigestion it is not because we are over acid but because we are under acid (a deficiency in hydrochloric acid). It is not a matter of too much acid, but a lack of the right one. People have to take these antacids because they do not understand cause and effect. We will cover this in the next chapter but for now we want to stress the fact that if we want to regain our health we have to change our acid conditions to alkaline. For those of you who presently have cancer or those of you who are fearful of getting it in the future, remember this fact: *malignant cells are acidic.* Eating the most nutritious food in the world will not heal us or maintain our health until we attain a proper acid/alkaline balance and maintain it.

Our bodies produce acid waste as a consequence of cell metabolism and these wastes are carried away through our eliminating channels. Excessive acidity is created when acids are produced faster than they are eliminated, or when alkaline chemicals are low, or when our eliminating systems are not functioning properly. Never forget that worry, fear and the other negative emotions produce acids in the body. That is why we spent so much time in the previous chapters regarding these emotions and their effects on our health. A hyperactive person is a sign of an increased effort by the body to eliminate acids so the pH may be maintained. When a person is sick (which means acidic) and refuses to take responsibility for themselves by not eating a diet high in the alkaline minerals such as calcium, silica, manganese, potassium, iodine and magnesium then there is no choice left but to go have the symptom treated. **All drugs accumulate in the body as acid waste, which further weakens the body.** The symptom may improve with the treatment but the body is left in a weakened condition.

There is so much more body chemistry than we have shared here; however, we have given you enough information to stimulate your interest should you choose to be responsible for your health. If you are presently sick or have a loved one who is, I would strongly urge you to contact a trained health-care professional who can help you maintain your proper body chemistry. It is unfortunate that young medical students are not being taught adequate body chemistry. This becomes more evident in the next chapter.

CHAPTER 12
HYDROCHLORIC ACID

Our bodies have two pH systems and each depends on the other. The one is the pH of the stomach, which is supposed to be acidic; and the other is the pH in our blood, which is supposed to be alkaline. Mass marketing has helped build a big business of selling ant-acids that destroy essential stomach acid. I mentioned in the previous chapter that people who suffer from acid indigestion do not have too much acid but they lack the proper one. Our bodies produce acids of fermentation when our HCL (hydrochloric acid) is low, and undigested food rots in our stomach and the result is acid indigestion. People then swallow antacids that further lower an already low stomach acid. At best this reduces the symptoms but the innocent patient has never been taught cause-and-effect. If our HCL is insufficient our digestion becomes incomplete which leads to cell starvation. Allopathic medicine treats this starvation as if it were a drug deficiency. The greatest majority of our elderly are low in hydrochloric acid because as we age our production of it declines. It is for this reason that supplementing our diet with it becomes essential if we want to maintain our vitality. All advertising for the antacids is geared toward the middle-aged or older and this should be a warning to us that indigestion is proportionate to our production of HCL.

I mentioned in the previous chapter that young medical students are not being taught proper body chemistry. An elderly pharmacist in our community showed me a 1923 medical book and in it contained eight columns showing the need for hydrochloric acid and what happens or does not happen when there is a lack of it. He then showed me a 1960 revised edition and it contained one paragraph on HCL. You can go to any library today and look at the latest edition of the Harvard school of medicine textbook and there is one sentence about hydrochloric acid. That sentence says hydrochloric acid is needed for digestion. This is a true statement in itself, however this is a little misleading. It is also needed to clean waste acids in the blood and lymph. Vitamin B-12 and folic acid are needed in the stomach to produce HCL. There are also several minerals needed in the stomach to produce it. HCL not only breaks down protein but it also digests bacteria and parasites as well. People who have adequate amounts of HCL have fewer infections. We increase our chances of getting pneumonia with insufficient HCL. When women have adequate HCL the breast fluid cells are normal, and if there is insufficient HCL there are usually pre-cancerous cells in the breasts. When we lack sufficient HCL we retain more carbon dioxide in the blood. When a person has a high carbon dioxide level he/she has lower oxygen content. Would a freethinking person with heart problems be interested in this information? Most people produce less HCL as they get older and many of them are taking antacids for misunderstood symptoms.

When the stomach is done processing what we eat it passes the substance into the first section of our small intestine where the pancreas washes it with antacids. The pancreas cannot do this without the alkaline elements. If this happens the small intestine will be slightly alkaline. So many people do not have the alkaline elements and that is why they develop ulcers near the valve that connect the stomach and the small intestine. When this function performs properly in the body, then one is on their way to maintaining a proper pH in the bloodstream. When the body (except for the stomach) is not slightly alkaline then that means it is living in an acid environment. Remember: if cells are healthy they are alkaline, and malignant cells are acidic; and one can never have healthy cells if they do not have the alkaline elements to achieve it. How many cancer patients are being told that they must eat more alkaline foods? They are not and for this reason we have more cancer today than ever before. No matter how well we eat or how much we exercise we will not be healthy until our pH is balanced properly.

Everyone knows the importance of calcium but few people know the importance of it beyond having strong bones. When calcium levels in the blood register too high it does not mean our calcium is too high but on the contrary it is low, or at least low in certain areas of the body. The reason calcium registers too high in the blood is because it is in transit from one place in the body to another. If we do not eat proper calcium or assimilate it, our brain will signal the body to transport it where it deems necessary. The calcium transported will come from our bones, teeth and gums. When we do not produce enough hydrochloric acid, calcium leaves the stomach taking other nutrients with it. Hydrochloric acid is critical for calcium absorption.

One of the main reasons that calcium is so important is that it alkalizes the body. Calcium attracts oxygen that is vital in combating degenerative diseases. This is a major reason why calcium assimilation is so critical and this does not happen when we lack hydrochloric acid. For one, cancer cannot live in an alkaline environment and healthy cells love it because of the oxygen carrying capacity of an alkaline environment. Cardiovascular disease is also precipitated by the lack of the proper calcium and or assimilation. People do not stop to ask why they get hardening of the arteries and not get hardening of the veins? Arteries have a layer of muscle around them that squeeze them to disburse blood to the body. Veins do not have this layer of muscle around them. Muscle tissue is more susceptible to acid than any other body tissue. If we do not have the proper calcium then lactic acid attacks our artery tissue. *This results in the artery building up a layer of cholesterol to protect itself. If this does not happen the lactic acid can cause us to hemorrhage. So you see, acid is the problem and not cholesterol.*

When we exercise we burn up more minerals and if we do not replace them at the same rate we burn them then lactic acid is the result. It is imperative we maintain our intake of alkaline minerals to maintain a proper pH in the body. Even if we have a proper intake of the alkaline minerals the body does not get total benefit from them when we lack hydrochloric acid.

Another mineral I want to briefly mention is zinc. We have such a low level of minerals in our soil here in America and one of the biggest reasons is because of all the synthetic supplements our agriculture industry uses. Next to nitrogen the mineral most depleted in our soil is zinc. I am mentioning this because zinc is necessary for our stomachs to produce HCL.

Zinc is necessary because it acts like a carrier to eliminate carbon dioxide from our body. Lack of zinc can lead to gray hair or loss of hair and it is also needed for the production of several sex hormones. Low levels of zinc can contribute to Crohn's disease, as well as rheumatoid arthritis, atherosclerosis, diabetes, upper respiratory infections, and low mental functions. Low levels of zinc can also lead to lower functioning of both the liver and the kidneys. Zinc is also for the healing of burns and wounds. Fatigue may be due to low levels of zinc. Cholesterol deposits are easier to dissolve with adequate levels of zinc. We mentioned above the mineral levels in the soil is very low, however, it is important to know alcohol reduces our zinc levels. Oral contraceptives in women will also reduce zinc levels. I mentioned above we need zinc to produce HCL. If you merely have adequate amounts of zinc for production of HCL then it is a guarantee you cannot have enough to avoid all the above maladies. **You can take an antacid for your bloated and gassy stomach, but you will be overlooking the warning the bloating is pointing to. If you only take something for the symptom instead of looking for the cause, then you could be prey to the above.**

If you think you can go out and buy synthetic zinc and take care of the problem you are sincerely deceived. You may be sincere but you still will be deceived.

There is another main point in maintaining a proper pH in the body I want to mention briefly. The body's homeostasis is working every second of every day to keep us in balance. So much of this is done through the glandular system which we discussed earlier in chapter two. When a person's homeostasis (the ability to regulate) declines they are headed for a disease and when the homeostasis ceases they die.

Another reason for maintaining a proper pH has to do with enzymes. Nothing we do while we are awake or sleeping happens without enzymes. Each of us has over 3000 different kinds of enzymes and each one performs its own task. Enzymes are protein molecules and there are millions of them in each of us. As we become more acidic our enzymatic functions decline proportionately, and when we become extremely acidic our enzymes start to die.

As mentioned before we cannot maintain a proper pH without adequate HCL. Raw foods have plenty of enzymes and since the American diet lacks adequate amounts of raw food we have fewer enzymes which make it more difficult for our bodies to maintain proper homeostasis. We cannot emphasize enough the fact that when a person is kept ignorant about cause and effect, he/she will be prey to various treatments for numerous symptoms.

When the two-pH systems in the body are correct then the other systems we have are more readily balanced. We will get into this in the next couple chapters.

CHAPTER 13
BALANCING OUR HORMONES

Sex hormone balancing is imperative to fight obesity and other diseases that are associated with aging. Since people are not being taught proper body chemistry they are in the dark as to why they develop male and/or female problems.

Let's begin with the females. There are over 750,000 hysterectomies a year in our country and estrogen dominance is the main problem. For years doctors have been prescribing estrogen to their female patients when they have any menopausal symptoms. The medical community in recent years has realized the dangers of excess estrogen, and today they our trying to balance estrogen with progesterone. They are using artificial progesterone (progestins) and those also have a list of negative side effects. The human body is incapable of producing enzymes to break down these synthetic hormones. Freethinking people know you cannot take artificial progestins to balance an artificial estrogen.

When you take natural progesterone you will not produce any secondary sex characteristics. It is imperative the progesterone you take is natural but it is more important that it is properly balanced with the estrogen. The body requires less progesterone if we can lower our estrogen which we will discuss later. Progesterone is so vital because it increases our libido, it enforces our thyroid function, it assists our body in the metabolism of fat for energy, and it helps us use oxygen better and helps to stimulate bone growth. Estrogen is not what we need to prevent osteoporosis; it is progesterone. Remember, humans can only break down two things, plants and animals. This understanding is vital to your health because once you understand this you will know that artificial progesterone cannot assist you in bone growth. This information is not hard to understand. What the medical profession wants us to believe is that health problems are complicated and we need them for solutions.

Hormone imbalances not corrected will make women susceptible to osteoporosis. Osteoporosis is a disorder of protein metabolism affecting bone structure. As we pointed out earlier insufficient HCL causes problems for digesting proteins. Our ability to secrete HCL is affected by estrogen. Estrogen imbalances are more likely to occur after surgery or at the onset of menopause. When estrogen levels drop the secretion of HCL drops also. I said it before and I will say it again: HCL is so critical to so many functions in the body. It is a shame doctors are not teaching their patients about something so vital to their health.

One male disease that is on the rise is prostate enlargement. Few people realize what the middle age spread is and/or what it is doing to them. It is a sign of estrogen dominance. Males and females take body fat and convert hormones into estrogen. The fatter we get the more estrogen dominant we become. What happens is, as we get heavier, estrogen levels in our prostate raise while at the same time our progesterone and testosterone lowers. When these last two hormones decline, it becomes a greater health risk to us than elevated estrogen. Testosterone is essential for life because it aids our carbohydrate metabolism, it has an effect in helping us lower our cholesterol, it helps us stabilize sugar, and it helps us with angina pain as well as other benefits.

The liver was created to remove any excess estrogen over and above the body's requirements. People in our country eat so much junk (we will discuss this in the next chapter) that their livers become overloaded so it cannot keep up with some of these functions. This is one of the main reasons so many ladies have trouble with sore breasts and other discomforts during their cycle. Some of the following vegetables have a property about them that will soak up extra estrogen: broccoli, Brussels sprouts, cabbage, bok choy, and cauliflower. When we lower our estrogen there is less stress to raise our progesterone.

There are more women developing female problems today than ever before and one myth is it is a condition that develops in midlife. Prior to midlife there are other signs or warnings that go unnoticed because we are not being taught how to read the body. Women are programmed to have menopausal conditions in midlife and have been programmed to take hormone replacement therapy (HRT) which is ingesting synthetic hormones. This practice continues even though it is common knowledge this puts the patient in greater danger for breast cancer later. If you have reproductive problems you will never get to the bottom of them until you realize you have an overall hormone imbalance. Most reproductive problems are the end result of previously undetected problems elsewhere in the body. Again, people are not being taught how to read this language.

Previously we discussed how prolonged stress clobbers the adrenals and the thyroid and this not only causes physical problems but psychological ones as well. Under stress hormone imbalances are created and the body sometimes overproduces certain hormones in an attempt to regain balance. The body also has the ability to convert sex hormones to stress hormones. If this process is done on a continual basis the person's reproductive system is challenged. This health condition is not as psychologically damaging to men as it is to women because men have male enhancement drugs available to them even though some men have experienced eye damage using some of them. If a doctor does not know how to improve your overall health he/she will give you a pill so you can at least perform. I have had two men tell me, after they took one of those pills for performance, everything turned blue. I could not believe they took the second one but people who do not think are always prey.

It is important to understand if one gland in the endocrine system is improperly functioning the rest of the glands in the system are disrupted as well. Understanding this is essential unless you are satisfied with only dealing with your symptoms.

When I said the other glands in the system are challenged as well, this definitely includes the thymus gland. Our overall health is directly proportionate to the health of our thymus gland. All the glands in this system are interrelated and this system is interrelated with everything else in the body. If you do not approach your health from this perspective, the only other choice you have left is to deal with symptoms. You will never have your hormones balanced as long as you are under continual stress and without peace of mind you will always be under stress. Stress can play itself out either mentally, emotionally or physically. That is why we spent time earlier explaining causes and solutions for troubled minds and emotions because without healthy minds and emotions we will never have healthy bodies.

There is more to balancing hormones than what I have listed here; however, if this information has stirred you to search deeper for answers for your own health problems then what I set out to do has been accomplished. The Internet and libraries are loaded with information regarding this. It takes time and energy to learn what you need to know for yourself and/or your loved ones who have health problems, but what you learn will become priceless. You cannot be watching television and playing computer games all the time and learn what you need to know to take care of yourself. *We should assume that the answers to our health are simple. It is merely a matter of searching for them.*

It was Shakespeare who said, "Of all knowledge, the wise and good seek most to know themselves." When you begin to know yourself you are in a position to begin regaining your health. This is wonderful but when you seek Him you are putting yourself in a position to have divine health.

CHAPTER 14
FOOD DECEPTION

Most Americans have an abundance of food to put in their stomachs; unfortunately, most of the food lacks vitality. People do not ask why we have full bellies and yet we have such a tremendous increase in degenerative diseases. Our agricultural industry and food processors provide us with food that is empty of any value and cannot enable us to sustain life. They make it taste so good by adding sugar, salt and other additives. This processed food will take care of our immediate need (hunger) but lacks the life to help us with tomorrow's need (healthy tissue and cells). If this were not true we would not have the weight problem we have in this country as well as such a tremendous growth in our hospital industry. The masses have been programmed to expect being overweight and sickly. We see heavy people having to use larger toilets than they used to. On the other hand we deny we have been programmed to be the same way later. Processed foods are stuffed with calories that are marked "enriched" on the packages. This is a scam because the foods are enriched with chemical or synthetic vitamins. The public is blind to this and they keep eating the same dead food. As a society we keep getting sicker; however, the public does not mind being slaves because they are being fed and entertained. Remember: humans do not have the ability to produce enzymes to break down anything other than plants or animals. Violating this natural law will only bring your own destruction.

I said in an earlier chapter it was not my purpose to go too deep into body chemistry but my focus was on tying the three-part person together. With that said, I would like to mention a couple chemistry misunderstandings we have about our bodies. We have been taught the body needs vitamin C but that is as far as it goes in the minds of most people. Vitamin C is essential for our entire cardiovascular system because it increases our ability to carry oxygen in the blood. This does not happen unless we have the whole vitamin C complex. The scam is most vitamin C sold is only ascorbic acid because the government has defined vitamin C as ascorbic acid. The truth is ascorbic acid is only part of the vitamin C family. When any vitamin is separated from its natural trace minerals and reduced to crystalline (made in a laboratory) form then the value to us as a food has been diminished. They have programmed the masses into believing that high potency is the key; but this is a bad misrepresentation because balance is the key. Ascorbic acid is only the antioxidant part of the family. This of course we need but it is only a fraction of the C family. Ignorance is expensive!! The public has been sold a bill of goods that is a crime of the utmost proportion.

While discussing vitamin C there is another point we would like to share. Our bodies have connective tissue that affects our nerves, organs, lymphatics, and blood vessels and reaches every cell. Collagen is the major component of connective tissue and you cannot build collagen without vitamin C. Our cardiovascular system cannot function without collagen. Collagen is also a major player in the motor center of our brains. You also need collagen for broken bones and wound healing. Scurvy is the last stage of our bodies not being able to produce collagen. Since collagen is produced on a daily basis we should supplement our diets with vitamin C. I personally take 3,000 mg. to 4,000 mg. of vitamin C daily. Anyone who has studied body chemistry knows it is an insult to think our bodies only need 400 mg. of C daily, the MDR established by the government. For heaven sake, do not think for a moment that you can buy synthetic C and be able to produce good connective tissue. It will not happen and if you try you will be mistaken. You may be sincere but nonetheless you will be mistaken. Do not forget, we only have the capability to break down plants and animals. Violating this natural law will bring on our own destruction if done on a daily basis.

Another example of this deception is vitamin E. Vitamin E is also classified by the government and they define it in terms of tocopherols. There are seven tocopherols of which Alpha tocopherol is one of them. The government rates vitamin E according to the amount Alpha tocopherol in the product. Like ascorbic C, Alpha tocopherol is only the antioxidant part of the vitamin E complex.

Vitamin E is important in the prevention of cancer and cardiovascular disease. It is beneficial in circulation, tissue repair, genital health, it helps promote blood clotting, helps reduce blood pressure, and aids in relaxing leg cramps. There are more benefits, but the point is, if you think you can put synthetic vitamin E in your system to help in the above, you are being deceived. Consumers believe they will be healthier taking the higher potency vitamins and that is what the manufacturers give them. The problem is that most of these products are minus the active ingredients; the natural cofactors. *The consumer asks and pays for bread but they are given crumbs.*

Another point of concern is the minimum daily requirements established by the government. There are 27 to 28 countries in the world that have higher minimum standards than we do in America. One in particular is folic acid. The medical community stresses the need for folic acid during pregnancy but what they claim is necessary is quite inadequate. Folic acid is measured in micrograms and the daily recommended requirement is 500 to 800 micrograms (mcg). In Europe they market it in milligrams and you can purchase it over-the-counter at 10 times the potency you can buy in America. We in America can still read so the medical community floods misrepresentation through the mass media to keep us confused.

The medical community claims 30 to 60 mgs is adequate amount of vitamin E for our daily requirement. It is amazing that my grandma had a heart attack in Canada and they immediately put her on 3600 mg of vitamin E. It is criminal what they do to Americans via the medical community. The problem is the medical community only use synthetic compounds in their research and you will develop problems if you ingest high doses of these elements. They will build up in your body (especially in the liver) but the body knows how to eliminate organic compounds because we have the capability to produce enzymes for that purpose. Medical research is tainted to benefit pharmaceuticals and not us. *If you do not know this then you are among the sheep and the sheep are always the prey.*

Another case in point we would like to mention is the MDR (minimum daily requirement) of the mineral iodine. The minimums established are set at a level just to keep you from getting something. The level of iodine established is merely enough to keep you from getting a goiter. Who in their right mind would want just enough iodine in their body to keep from getting a goiter? I know we discussed iodine in Chapter seven when we were discussing the thyroid but here we are talking about the mineral, and not the gland. Iodine is necessary in other parts of the body such as: the pituitary, the liver, the gallbladder, reproductive organs in the male and female, the brain, the heart, the hair and scalp, the veins and arteries, and the joints. If you only ingest enough iodine to keep you from getting a goiter you could become prey to the above maladies.

We are talking about food iodine here, not the radioactive form. Food iodine has been given to patients thousands of times more than the minimum daily requirement and found to be very safe. Again, if all you know about the chemistry requirements of our bodies, which have been approved by the FDA, then the degenerative diseases that plague mankind are waiting for you. If and when a doctor runs some test on you, and finds your thyroid hormones to be low then he/she more than likely will prescribe a synthetic thyroid hormone. This may alleviate some of the former symptoms of a low functioning thyroid; however, this does nothing to raise the body's need for adequate iodine to eliminate some of the other symptoms because of an iodine deficiency. When iodine levels become low it begins to affect our memory, we are susceptible to becoming more tired, we can experience menstrual problems, our muscles can become weak, we can become more irritable, begin experiencing muscle cramps, maybe have elevated cholesterol, begin experiencing dry skin, and our nails start becoming more brittle.

This is not a complete list of symptoms because of the lack of iodine. It is merely our intent to point out should you have any of the above symptoms you should have the freedom to seek out a professional who is trained to help with your body chemistry. I just mentioned this is a partial list of symptoms and our libraries and the Internet are full of information for those seeking the truth. It is exciting to seek truth because it is the only thing that will set you free. I am sharing this information about iodine with you, only to point out the minimums established for our health is a farce. Common sense tells you if we spend more money in America compared to all other countries for healthcare, and there are 29 to 30 countries in the world whose citizens are healthier than we are, then something has gone awry.

I want to touch on another subject that has become center stage since the passing of former President Reagan and that is Alzheimer's disease. In order to bring out one aspect of Alzheimer's disease I feel I have to go back and repeat myself on a previous principal. We pointed out when acid penetrates the muscles around the arteries we can hemorrhage if the arteries tear. The brain then sends in some cholesterol to patch up the damage so the tear does not happen. Cholesterol is not the problem it is our friend. Acid is the problem! Our bodies have so many backup systems and I would like to point out another one. If our arteries are in danger of tearing, in addition to the cholesterol being sent in, the brain sends in extra calcium as a healer. When our bodies do not have adequate calcium in our blood to help strengthen the walls of the arteries then the body will pull calcium out of our teeth and gums to do the job. This process will save our lives; however, if we continually use our backup system then the hard calcium will make our arteries hard. The problem is we do not want the same calcium in our artery walls that is in our teeth and bones. As I just said, this will save us temporarily but over time it will make our artery walls harder which is major in developing hardening of the arteries. In addition, we certainly do not want the same calcium that makes good hard bones to get into our brains or our brain will calcify.

We have several kinds of calcium in the body, and we need them all to be healthy. Each one of them has a specific purpose. This process (transporting calcium from one point to another) is happening in most people because of all the inorganic calcium people are buying. If you are buying calcium (or any other supplement) that our bodies cannot manufacture enzymes to break them down then the supplement is useless.

Silica is another mineral in the body that has many uses, one of which is to keep our elasticity proper. **Our bodies have the ability to take existing silica and convert it into calcium.** The brain chooses the consequences of living without enough silica verses lacking proper calcium. This brings us to Alzheimer's disease. There have been many studies that have implicated aluminum with Alzheimer's. So many Americans are ingesting aluminum on a daily basis, whether it is in their drinking water, beverages in aluminum cans or wrapping their food in aluminum foil. **We now know that silica can drastically reduce aluminum in the body. As we just mentioned we have such a lack of silica because we lack the proper calcium.**

Our Father in all His wisdom knew the end from the beginning and provided contingencies for everything. There is more to Alzheimer's disease than a lack of silica; however, this should be enough information for you to starting searching for yourself and/or your loved ones. As in any disease, balance must be achieved and maintained. We will never make any progress in any of these diseases until we grasp the truth that the human body was never intended for any inorganic compounds.

What I have shared with you in regard to these vitamins and minerals is a tip of the iceberg compared to all the other information available concerning all the nutrients we need. Most health food stores have a library of information for those who are seeking the truth. This is quite the opposite of sitting in front of the television expecting to be entertained. Learning the truth takes time and discipline but once you start to learn, then it will begin to set you free. We have to learn what we need to eat; however, it is equally important to learn what not to eat. At this point I want to bring up another issue that is so important in maintaining or regaining our health.

We were created a mineral first, then a vegetable, and lastly an animal. If we choose to develop our spiritual senses that is wonderful; however, whether you develop them or not you will always be those first three as long as you are sucking air in this life. All of our vegetables are high in some minerals and low in others. If we do not eat a variety of them we will have an overabundance of some minerals we need and be deficient in others. It does not make any difference if you understand the need of minerals or not, becoming deficient in them will spiral your health downward. We need the minerals because of their reproductive value. When we eat hybrid grains and vegetables we are not ingesting necessary life producing substances. A point at hand is: if we go out in a field and find a sunflower plant, we eat the seed and not the plant. If the seed can reproduce itself it can reproduce life in us.

When Americans started eating all the hybrid food, cancer went sky high. This is because open pollinated grain and vegetables have vitamin B-17 in them but the hybrids have next to none. Vitamin B-17 is the cancer-fighting vitamin. What has developed is a multi-national company has a division that builds a plant to produce the hybrid seeds, and then later that same company has another division which builds a plant in another location that makes chemotherapy to put in people after they get cancer from eating food that has no vitamin B-17. The company makes money at both ends.

On top of this, food producers are radiating our food. Everyone knows radiation weakens our immune system. Most adults have seen pictures of the people in Japan taken after we dropped the atomic bomb on them, and how burned they were. Yet people will eat food that has been treated with the same substance. Remember: sheep are cute and very sweet but boy are they stupid. The reason the food producers are radiating our food is supposedly those eating their products (notice I said products and not food) will get less infections, etc. If we have enough HCL in our stomachs then any larva or bacteria ingested will be digested before it gets to our small intestine. It is sad that our pre-med students are being kept in the dark about such a vital point.

A similar issue is Americans eating genetically modified food (GMO) when there are countries in Europe who refuse to import our GMO foods. GMO seeds were modified to resist pesticides and herbicides. It seems the Europeans are less neutered than we Americans. We will explain neutered in the conclusion of the book. We cannot produce enzymes to break down those food products and unless you understand this principle and apply this knowledge you will suffer with the rest of the sheep.

Eating white processed sugar is detrimental to the health of consumers; however, it is very healthy for the hospital industry. Eating refined sugar throws off the body's homeostasis that results in a variety of significant consequences. The following is a partial list of some of those consequences.

1. Sugar can suppress the immune system.
2. Sugar can cause hyperactivity, anxiety and concentration difficulties.
3. Sugar can elevate triglycerides.
4. Sugar can cause liver and kidney damage.
5. Sugar interferes with absorption of calcium and magnesium.
6. Sugar is a major factor in all cancers.
7. Sugar promotes tooth decay and periodontal disease.
8. Sugar increases the risk of crohn's disease and colitis.
9. Sugar contributes to gallstones and kidney stones.
10. Sugar contributes to hemorrhoids and varicose veins.
11. Sugar contributes to osteoporosis.
12. Sugar can change the structure of protein which interfere with the protein being absorbed.
13. Sugar can cause food allergies.
14. Sugar contributes to diabetes.
15. Sugar contributes to cardiovascular disease.
16. Sugar contributes to emphysema.
17. Sugar contributes to free radical formation in the bloodstream.
18. Sugar lowers the ability of enzymes to function (remember: we cannot digest without enzymes).
19. Sugar can contribute to fluid retention.
20. Sugar can contribute to constipation.
21. Sugar can contribute to hypertension.
22. Sugar can cause headaches, including migraines.
23. Sugar can cause depression.
24. Sugar can increase bacterial fermentation in the colon.
25. Sugar can increase the risk of Alzheimer's disease.

This is only a partial list; however, it is adequate for any freethinking person to know the health risk to his/her health. A lot of our senior citizens remember the sugar shortage and rationing during World War II. During that time there was less illness because there was less sugar available. Why are people so blind that they cannot see the handwriting on the wall? I mentioned in the above list that sugar could contribute to hyperactivity in children and add this to the fact the masses have been led to believe what used to be normal childhood behavior is now a mental illness that requires drugs to treat. Parents have been numbed down so much they accept the fact it is wrong to spank their children but, it is satisfactory to give them drugs for behavioral problems that hurt the liver. This whole scenario is insane. One out of 30 of our children are on these drugs and this is a disgrace to our society. The high consumption of sugar in this country has become the perfect crime because it makes everyone eventually a prospect for prescription drugs. *Remember: no one is ever sick because they have a lack of drugs in them. I mentioned earlier most people want to eat what they want to eat, when they want to eat it, harbor all the bad feelings against everyone who has ever hurt them, then these people become prey to the drug companies.*

While discussing sugar we want to bring out another aspect of cancer. Look at the diagram below.

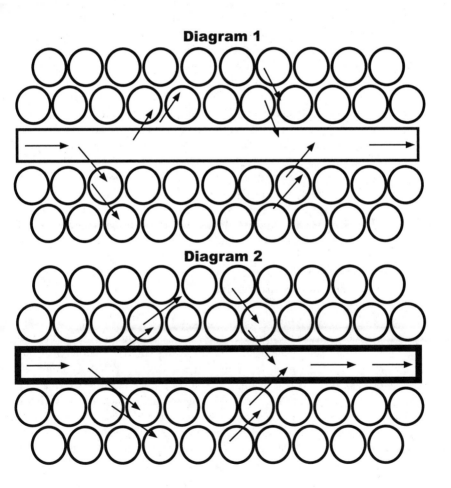

Let's look at diagram 1 in two ways. The two lines in the center represent a hallway in a hotel. The first row of circles next to the line represents the room where the bed is and the second row of circles represents the bathrooms. The arrows on the left represent the flow of people going from the hallway to the first room and then into the bathroom. This is pictured just the opposite by the arrows on the right side of the diagram representing people leaving the rooms. Let us suppose all hallways; all the rooms including the bathrooms are jammed with people. If a fire alarm goes off the people in the rooms cannot begin to enter the hallway until the people in the hallway clear out. The people in the bathrooms cannot begin clearing out until the people in the rooms begin clearing out into the hallways.

Now look at the diagram, the space between the lines is our blood stream and the row of circles next to it is lymphatic fluid and the third row is our cells. To clean the body anywhere, you must clean the bowel first, then the blood and finally make sure you get the blood where it needs to go. No matter what part of your body is sick you are doing nothing for yourself but putting on bandages until your blood is clean. This is why getting your pH balanced is so critical. This chapter is titled Food Deception so I want to illustrate how the above plays out in our daily lives.

When a cell begins to get weakened it will discard the weakened part and replace it with new material. The cell swims through the lymphatic fluid to get close to a capillary to get the proper substances from our blood to replace the old. What happens is, through small openings in the capillary the cells get whatever they need from our blood and after that happens it swims away. Here is where the problem begins. We need to understand composition of blood before we go any farther. Our blood is over ninety percent water. We eat protein and from these proteins the body makes additional proteins, which are referred to as blood proteins. The balance of the blood is minerals, etc. When we do not drink enough water then the percent of water in our blood will drop and the percent of blood protein goes up. Since the protein is thicker than water this makes our blood thicker. Doesn't it make sense to drink more water if your blood is too thick than to take a drug that has the same substance that kills rats?

Thickened blood now becomes a major problem. When the holes in the capillaries open to let food substances through to feed the cells, sometimes the little holes open up too much and some blood proteins escape through the openings. _This is not a problem if the lymph fluid can remove it fast enough._ When it cannot, then trouble begins. Now look at diagram 2. You see a thick layer next to the blood wall, which represents a build up of blood proteins outside the capillaries. This is a major cause of cancer, and the reason is when a cell needs to reach the capillaries it cannot because of the thick wall that separates them. If the cell cannot get oxygen from our blood stream (there is a lot of oxygen in water), then the glucose (sugar) in our little cell will start to ferment without oxygen. This process is why so many people have yeast, which is a breakdown that leads to cancer. _Cells without oxygen_ _will turn cancerous._ The question that should be asked then, why do the openings in the capillaries open too wide? There are five substances people consume that produce the problem: sugar, salt, caffeine, alcohol and nicotine.

There also is an emotional aspect that needs to be addressed. In a home where there is a lot of negative directed from the parents to the children, the same problems can occur. An example of this is when a parent screams at a child: "How could you be so dumb?" or "How stupid can you be?" or "I am so ashamed of you!!" These types of questions or statements will shock the openings up just as will the five food substances mentioned. This is why it is imperative to look at the person and not just the body.

Children or babies will let you know what is going on inside a home if you know how to listen to them. I was called to a home where a baby had been crying for five days. The parents met me at the door when I arrived and you could hear the baby crying from the other end of the house. I asked the parents if everything was okay with them and they both replied yes. They then proceeded to lead me back to the bedroom where the baby was. I looked down in the crib and said "Hey, little one, are you upset with me?" The baby kept crying so I said "Is everything okay with you and mommy?" The baby continued so I said "Is everything okay with you and daddy?" Instantly, the crying stopped. I looked over to the dad and he dropped his head. He had been yelling at the mom and the baby responded accordingly. I placed this incident here to show how our emotions affect us just as much as the food we eat. You can be sure that baby had been producing a lot of acid for those five days.

While discussing food deception there are three products sold as food we consume that create havoc in so many people. One is monosodium glutamate (MSG) to which over 20,000,000 Americans react negatively. George R. Schwartz, M.D. wrote a book called IN BAD TASTE that goes to great length explaining the result of ingesting this product. If you suffer from asthma, diarrhea, headache, hyperactivity, heart irregularities, muscle aches, incontinence, chest pain, dizziness, nausea, rashes, mood swings, hot flashes, shortness of breath, stomach cramps, depression, I would recommend reading his book or you can look on the internet. Type in monosodium glutamate, then click on MSG and other glutamates, then click on monosodium glutamate newswired.net and you will get a complete list of symptoms associated with MSG.

The second product we want to look at is aspartame. If you suffer from the symptoms of fibromyalgia, spasms, shooting pains, numbness in your legs, cramps, vertigo, headaches, tinnitus, joint pain, depression, anxiety, blurred vision, or memory loss I would strongly recommend you go to the internet and type in aspartame to search out what this product does in the body and why. If you do you will get a more detailed list of associated problems connected to consuming aspartame. Not having a computer is no excuse because your friends or local library have one.

The third product we want to mention is corn syrup or high fructose corn syrup. High fructose corn syrup is a favorite among food processors because it is cheap to produce and it has a long shelf life against crystallizing. Go to the internet and type in high fructose corn syrup and click on the murky world of high fructose corn syrup. Another site to click on is the Weston A. Price Foundation "The double danger of high fructose corn syrup." Diabetes has increased seven fold over the last 50 years and you wonder when people will wake up. To so many people doctors are considered gods, but it is amazing to me how the gods have developed beta blockers, calcium blockers, and fat blockers but have not developed sugar blockers. If they would the medical industry would collapse. We are fast becoming a nation of diabetics and no one is teaching our youth how to avoid this plague.

Something equally as bad as our food processors using these three substances in our food supply is the congressmen who allow it. We elect our congressmen and senators to represent us and they are supposed to be public servants. Even though our officials have all been made aware of these three food substances and the side affects, they allow them to be used. They bow to the pressure of big money and if they do not they will not be reelected. They basically sell their souls to keep their positions of power. They compromise their constituents who voted them in office.

If all this information is new to you and you want to learn, it is easy to do so if your heart is open. Only a hardened heart will not consider the information given in the above paragraphs. Of all the discipline among God's children, rebellion seems to be the hardest. Ps.68-6 "the rebellious dwell in a dry land." *If you are sick you are in a dry land.* If you are rebellious you have the nature of a bull. Bulls use their strength and aggressiveness to gratify themselves. A bull cannot serve because it cannot submit and it cannot submit because it refuses to be broken. If you are rebellious then you will refuse to listen to anyone and you will show no interest in what we have shared with you. The only alternative then is to become the prey. You may not care now, but you will remember this just before they saw your leg off when you have diabetes or when they are giving you chemotherapy when you have cancer. Remember: the sheep are led to the slaughter.

In the next chapter we will discuss how our body chemistry has such an effect on our weight. We said earlier it is not our intent to share too much body chemistry; however, we feel this information is necessary because being an obese nation affects the health of all of us. If you are not one of the obese ones you still are affected by the general health of the nation.

CHAPTER 15
WEIGHT AND DIETING

There is more misinformation, scams and confusion regarding weight loss than other health issues because there is such a demand for solutions to our weight problems. **Most of the good information does not work because people want a silver bullet. Most of the false information does not work because it violates human nature.** If you are sincere about losing weight and being healthy then you must stay disciplined and focused. If you cannot imagine it then it will never become a reality to you. You must have the victory in your mind first before you go any farther. I mentioned in the previous chapter most foods are not foods at all but are merely nonfoods produced by food processors. The more we eat these empty foods the more we crave them and they end up becoming fat. To lose weight we must have a sustainable program that must include us getting out of the mindset we have to starve ourselves to achieve our goal. If you eat food that is right for you then you can eat as much as you want and not gain any weight. Notice I said food that is right for you because not everyone should be eating the same food. A list of recommended reading concerning this will be at the end of the book.

To have a stable workable program for losing weight we must get out of the mindset that fat is the problem. We have all known people who have died very young who had no fat on them at all. *Any and all degenerative diseases are because of a nutritional lack.* People have been eating low fat or no fat food, as long as it has been recommended; yet we have more heart problems today than ever before. This is a warning to free thinkers but definitely not to gullible people.

The issue is not fat or carbohydrates but bad fat and bad carbohydrates. Bad fats are synthetically made fats such as hydrogenated or partially hydrogenated. To make margarine they take soy, corn or cottonseed oil and extract it from the grain. They then take this and mix it in a vat that contains nickel oxide and cook it at very high-temperature. This mixture has a poor consistency so they add emulsifiers and starch. This mixture is not very appealing so they bleach it. The substance is now hydrogenated which means they spray it with hydrogen gas under tremendous pressure (at 400 degrees). This process will change the liquid oil into a semi solid solution. At this point it is still not ready to go to market. Emulsifiers are forced into the oil keeping the water from separating out, and then it must be mechanically forced together, or homogenized. They now add starch to increase consistency. Next they add dyes, color and flavorings to make it taste like something that it is not. Once they add preservatives it is now ready for consumption. I tell people butter is better for them than margarine especially if the butter is made from raw milk. Our liver was created to break down animal fats but it was not created to break down dyes, detergents and solvents. It does not make any difference if you know and understand His natural laws (eating the oils we were created to break down) or understand them and violate them, the consequences are the same. Since the liver cannot break down these hardened oils they are then deposited somewhere in the body and will only cause havoc.

Another point of concern when consuming these heavier oils is they require more oxygen to break them down. This makes our breathing heavier because the lungs are working harder to get more oxygen in our bodies. Our heart will start pumping harder because of the additional lung activity. Also people who consume the bad fats are making themselves immune deficient. Consumers are led to believe by eating these oils they are making their hearts healthier but in reality they are making themselves more vulnerable to cancer because of the immune system being weakened. Common sense tells you these bad oils suppress the immune system because the medical community really stresses the use of these oils on any patient who has had a transplant. A person who has an immunosuppression disease (such as multiple sclerosis, psoriasis, rheumatoid arthritis, etc.) may experience relief from eating these oils, however; anything that suppresses the immune system will make you vulnerable to cancer. You can believe who and what you want, but the bottom line is that 100 years ago people were eating lard and butter and the cancer rate was 1/5 of what it is today.

All cancer research is focused on how to treat the disease instead of studying healthy people and find out why they do not get this disease. If you are victim of all the misinformation concerning cancer then you will be one who sends your hard earned money for research that is focused on the effect and not the cause. There is more to cancer than consuming bad oils but this a major player. Never forget, if you eat and live like the masses then how the masses end up will be your fate.

I put the problem of bad oils in this chapter because we are discussing weight loss. Any oil that cannot be broken down becomes problematic in trying to lose weight. I said in a previous paragraph that processed oils are treated at 400 degrees and it takes a minimum of 350 degrees to break them down. Since our bodies are 98 degrees it is impossible to break these oils down.

People who retain water or swell are dehydrated. It is imperative that we drink more water to make the body stop retaining it. **We must have an abundance of water because water is necessary to metabolize fat.** So overweight people need more water than thin people because they have larger metabolic loads. When we put ourselves on a program to lose weight we must understand that our body processes more waste, resulting from the breakdown of fat, and we need extra water to carry this waste out.

Even though water is critical to our health we must understand not all water is water. Fluoridated water can cause some people to gain weight. Drinking water that has been treated with chlorine and fluoride can hinder us from losing weight because those chemicals enter the body and slow down iodine utilization. We need iodine for our thyroid gland to function properly. In addition, fluoride inhibits enzymes in the body; consequently, heavy people merely store food, they do not burn it. Some people do not understand why when they drink diet sodas they do not lose weight. That is because they are all made out of fluorinated water. Another issue to be addressed is that too much copper in the tissues can slow down your metabolism. Copper in our plumbing can leach into the water which causes this problem. A lot of the flavored water drinks are high in copper so we do not want to drink too much of these when trying to lose weight.

The problem with most diet plans is they can make you very tired. Common sense and balance is the key. The latest craze is the high protein and low carbohydrate diet. This works for most people for a season but sooner or later they will begin cheating to keep their energy up. You can talk to a dieter all day long about not eating certain foods but once his energy levels go down so low it does not matter. Losing energy will ruin the best of diets. It is totally erroneous information that carbohydrates are not good for you. It depends on what form they are in. Processed carbohydrates are devastating when you are trying to lose weight, but without eating some carbohydrates you will not have the necessary energy to burn fat. It takes a lot of energy to burn fat so to the extent that you eat carbohydrates are you capable of generating energy from burning fat. When you cannot get energy from your fat then the body can break down any muscle and convert as much as 50% of it into glucose for energy. This is why so many dieters begin having saggy skin, isn't it very attractive? To reach your long-term weight objectives, be sure to include some complex carbohydrates in your diet so you have them to burn for energy.

There is another issue I want to share here for a moment. We have had in our business for several years a product called conjugated linoleic acid (CLA). This product has a property about it that helps reduce body fat at the same time increases lean muscle mass. Beef is high in this nutrient and this may be one of the reasons so many people have had success on the Atkin's and South Beach diets. Something interesting was uncovered recently and it was that beef from Australia had 400% more of this nutrient than American beef. Everything else being equal, people in Australia will have an easier time losing weight than Americans. I do not know the practices in our commercial feed lots that differ from those in Australia. There is more to our weight problem in America than people being lazy, although this greatly contributes to the problem as well.

There is 25% of our population who are sensitive to monosodium glutamate (MSG). I know I mentioned MSG in the previous chapter but it is important to understand how this product affects some people's weight. If you are having trouble losing weight I would strongly suggest you go to the internet and type in MSG. Then click on truthinlabeling.org. and then click obesity epidemic. If you have not been exposed to this cover up, as to how this product actually makes it harder for you to lose weight, this information will make you livid. MSG is an addictive substance and the food processors know this. They know the more you eat this substance the more of their product you will want to eat. While you are on this web sight it might behoove you to read the potential problem of losing weight when you consume aspartame (Nutra Sweet, Equal and others). The government, on the surface, claims to show interest in our weight epidemic, yet sanctions products that intensify the problem. It is imperative for you to be responsible for your health and the health of your loved ones. The information in this paragraph attests to this.

I cannot stress enough the value of using common sense when trying to lose weight. You cannot violate natural healing laws and sustain yourself for any length of time. I said earlier that we should not all be eating the same diet. We must learn what our body type and metabolism is. There are people who have tried a particular diet and when it worked they thought everyone should do the same. That is not correct. For instance, some people are better off being vegetarians but this is not true for everyone. If your heritage is from northern Europe (they ate a lot of fatty fish through the years) then you will be able to metabolize fat better than those whose heritage is from a tropical climate. If you take a person whose heritage is from the tropics (who ate more fruits) and try to feed them a lot of fatty foods you will slowly kill them. The same principle applies to people who come from a long line of meat eaters, because if you try to make them vegetarians you will slowly do them in as well. This is because people who have a heritage of meat eaters have a digestive system geared to producing more hydrochloric acid.

My wife is one of those people and she can only go about 4 to 5 days without meat. When she wakes up in the morning and looks like a lioness when someone is threatening her cubs then I know it is time get her some meat. I run out to the freezer and grab a frozen steak, whereupon I open up the bedroom door and throw it in quickly and slam the door. After all the growling has stopped then I know it is safe to open the door. That act of kindness (actually it is merely learning her body chemistry and needs) on my part turned her from a lioness to a kitty. Again, if you want to lose weight (without compromising your health) we must learn our individual requirements. It is not important what someone else needs. It is your goal regarding weight loss and health you are to be concerned with.

To lose weight you begin by eating less and exercising more. To drink a lot of diuretic teas without changing your diet will only be detrimental to your health. There are no quick fixes! To lose weight you must set your goals but make sure they are attainable; otherwise, you will get discouraged and quit. It is fine to eat protein but it must be balanced with the complex carbohydrates, eating plenty of vegetables and some fruit. It is possible to lose weight without exercising if you balance your body chemistry right; however, you will never firm up without it. Common sense dictates that you should exercise to help reach your goal. Do yourself a favor and find someone who has been trained to help you balance your body chemistry; otherwise, at best you will be in a hit or miss proposition. *If you balance your body chemistry so you can lose weight you will find the benefits are insurmountable. When body chemistry is balanced right, degenerative diseases will more than likely bypass you later in life.* Please read this last sentence again!! The very best to you! Remember, you do not have to be a rocket scientist to do this.

CHAPTER 16
ALLERGIES

An allergy is a response by the body's immune system to a substance that normally is not harmful. I am not going into all the "what to do" or "what to avoid" if you and or your loved ones suffer from allergies. There is an abundance of this information available already on the market; however, that said, I would like to point out a couple of facts important to allergy sufferers.

As pointed out earlier our immune system is our first line defense mechanism in keeping us healthy <u>and love is the most important factor in keeping our immune system working at an optimal level.</u> The immune system is to identify anything foreign in our body and make appropriate responses so these foreign substances become harmless to us. It is imperative we develop and maintain a healthy immune system if we want to deal with any allergies we may have. With that said, I would like to mention some body chemistry regarding our immune system.

White blood cells, some are T-cells, recognize and begin destroying viruses, bacteria, fungus, and cancer cells. B-cells are another group of white blood cells for manufacturing antibodies. Earlier I mentioned the spleen has a role in our immune system. The lymph system cleans us at the cellular level and it also cleans the fluid between the cells. The lymph system cleans and drains waste material.

People with allergies usually have higher counts of white cells verses the non-allergy people. Phosphorous is present in white cells, and wheat has an overabundance of phosphorous; consequently, allergy sufferers should cut way back on wheat consumption and some even need to eliminate it all together. Both the lungs and the kidneys rid the body of old phosphorous and if phosphorous is over consumed the lungs and kidneys become challenged.

Another point we want to interject concerning allergies and the immune system involves birth. When a mother is giving birth naturally, the baby is coming down the birth canal with the mouth open. The mother's vagina has a substance the baby ingests (it is taken in through the open mouth) as it passes through. This substance has a powerful immune system stimulant. There are circumstances when the mother's safety would be at risk during a natural birth and a caesarian birth is a better option; however, everything else being equal, a natural birth has its advantages concerning the baby's immune system. Colostrum (the first substance out of the mother's breast after birthing) is another immune system stimulant. It is a known fact mothers who birth their babies naturally and breast feed them will have children with fewer allergies than those mothers who do not.

We become more prone to infectious diseases without our immune system operating properly; however, we can also become ill if our immune system over reacts or directs its functions to a substance inappropriately. This gets into all the autoimmune disorders.

It is amazing man can go to the moon but he cannot figure out how to cure the common cold. The cold is the cure! It is the body trying to rid itself of excess waste. Trying to suppress the waste will only complicate your life later. This is attested to the fact allergies represent the body's desperate attempt to rid itself of waste and foreign substances. Taking suppressant medications will challenge your health as the waste continues to create havoc within your body. When any waste is held in the body, the place the waste settles becomes weaker which will lead to a chronic degenerative disease.

I cannot emphasize enough the need to look at the person and not just the body if you want a healing. It is a given that everyone has inherited certain physiological weaknesses. If you compound emotional weight on top of those weaknesses the body will cave in. Let's use a child with an inherent weakness in his/her respiratory system as an example. The child normally will develop more colds than usual which the parents treat with an over the counter suppressant medication. In a home where the parents fight a lot some of the children develop nervous irregular bowel habits. Over time the toxic residue from the cold medication will settle at the weakest point in the body. When constipation develops any excess toxins not passed out of the bowel will be reabsorbed into the bloodstream which will settle in the weakest point. In this case, it will be in the respiratory system. This child will go from simple colds, if the situation is not corrected, to bronchial colds, and then if not corrected can lead to allergies.

Parents with children may want to reevaluate their smoking. I do not judge people who do certain things because I have not walked in their shoes; however, there is something else parents who have children with allergies or other respiratory problems should be aware of. Our first line of defense against airborne particles is our tonsils and adenoids. These two are part of our lymphatic system and require the mineral sulphur to operate at an optimal level. Secondary smoke (as well as other airborne chemicals) will take sulphur out of the body. When these two do not filter out harmful airborne particles the lungs react to them.

To help remove waste from our bodies it is imperative to exercise. This increases the strength of our respiratory system which enables us to bring in more oxygen. The lower the oxygen content in the body coupled with a build up of toxic waste will challenge our health. Years ago kids worked all day in the sun and were a lot healthier than kids today. Today parents are being taught how to have organized activities indoors to keep the children from supposed harmful sunrays.

Just recently it was on the national news child asthma is up 10-fold and childhood diabetes is skyrocketing. When will parents wake up? Ignorance is not bliss!

Chapter 17
WATER AND AIR

There are two other aspects of our bodies' requirements for existence and they are water and air.

Municipalities purify our water by adding fluorine and chlorine to kill any bacteria and other harmful substances. The problem is all the chemicals running into our streams and rivers from fields are still in the water you drink. This certainly is not new news evidenced by the tremendous purifying water systems sold in our country. More people than not are installing reverse osmosis systems which are great, but we personally drink distilled water. In reverse osmosis systems the debris is taken out of the water, but by distilling the water you are taking the water out of the debris. In response to critics of drinking distilled water, they claim there is no food value left after distilling, and they are correct. However, the minerals in community water systems and wells are all inorganic. Our bodies do not function properly on inorganic compounds.

One of the advantages of drinking distilled water is it has a much greater capacity to clean our bodies. We personally take organic supplements, so drinking distilled water is not a concern to us. One thing I would not do is drink distilled water out of a store. It is poured into brand new plastic jugs and the chemicals in the plastic will leach into the water. We subscribe to several publications and one of them ran a comparative study of the different distilling systems and Waterwise, Inc. out of Florida was recommended. The telephone number is 1-800-874-9028. The publication that recommends them and myself, do not receive anything for recommending this company. If a company treats you right, it is our responsibility to share it with others. We have bought several of their distillers over the years, which we gave most of them to friends, and not one of them had a complaint about this company. Unless we drink the purest water possible our health cannot be maintained at an optimal level.

Air is an essential substance of life. For people to live they breathe about 2500 gallons of air per day. Not all air is the same. Polluted air does not have as much negative ions as pure air. In enclosed environments, such as homes and work places, the positive ions increase. Drapes, synthetic carpets, electronic equipment, and other objects in our homes and work places remove negative ions from the air. Negative ions attract molecules of toxic materials and drop them to the floor. The higher the negative ions in the air the better we feel. After a lightening storm the air is saturated with negative ions and that is why we feel better being outside after a storm. Nature has other means of creating negative ions: fires, waterfalls, ocean surf meeting the air, etc. For this reason we have several ion generators in our home and one for the car because anyone who breathes air with too many positive ions in it will be more susceptible to colds, flu, allergies, and being tired. You can learn more about ions by contacting the University of the Trees Press, P.O. Box 66, Boulder Creek, California 95006. Ask for "You are what you Breathe" by Robert Massy, Ph. D.

Physical objects affect the ions in our atmosphere but there is an emotional issue we also want to point out. When Adam and Eve were created they were balanced perfectly. After the fall their children and all of mankind since have been born overcharged on the positive side. When we get angry, and do not deal with it, then we are generating a body that produces a more positive charge. The body produces more and more until it finally blows up (anger released) and then the person feels better. Then the process starts all over again. Every time this happens the body is releasing a positive charge in the atmosphere. The universe operates the same as we do. Each one of us is a small universe within ourselves connected electrically to the bigger one. If and when the earth's atmosphere has too much positive charge, it releases it the same way people do. A storm is generating negative ions (created by friction) which balance the positive and negative ions. As in us, there is calm after the storm.

When our country left our Christian heritage and moved to humanism, and people are not held accountable for their actions, the morals have decayed. The same degree morals decline, crime increases proportionately. The degree of crime increase in our country since the advent of humanism is indicative of the level our morals have declined. *Every time we sin we emit positive ions in the atmosphere.* The point is, as the morals of a nation decline, weather patterns are altered. People think if they violate someone else's rights and do not get caught, they have gotten away with it. The above disproves that logic. We never get away with anything for any length of time.

I want to say again I believe in medicines, but the ones that have worked since the beginning of time. Water and air are definitely two of these medicines, but they must be in the purest form for us to operate at optimal levels.

CHAPTER 18
POLITICS AND OUR HEALTH

Briefly we want to look at several political situations and how they eventually play out regarding our health.

Recently a judge made a decision that United Airlines does not have to pay the flight attendants their retirement most of them had worked years to accumulate. I am surprised that judge is still alive. The bigger picture becomes obvious as a precedent has been set. What is going to keep General Motors, Ford or any other major corporation from doing the same? We were watching the national news that night and a United Airlines male employee had just been told he would not be receiving his pension. He said he was really "P----- Off!" Any and every other person in any industry who has worked loyally for their employer and then find out the company would not honor its word would make anyone livid. This situation at United Airlines is a tip of the iceberg compared to what else is coming in our country.

It is not my intent to discuss political decisions, only how they affect our lives regarding health. The employee who was upset, and justifiably so, will have his thyroid hammered if he stays angry for any length of time. As we pointed out earlier, the thyroid controls so much heart function. When he retires, without the pension he counted on, there will be increased financial stress on him and his wife, if he is married. The stress put on him can weaken his adrenals, which can increase the chances of developing either diabetes, cancer, heart problems or arthritis. If this employee stays angry his health can spiral downward because the anger is controlling him. No one could fault him for this, but nonetheless, he pays the price measured by the status of his physical, mental and emotional well being.

A man I recently talked to makes honey for a living. He said the market dropped off because of cheap honey coming in from China. When we were young it was something to be proud of that we were feeding so much of the world. Today Communist China helps feed us. It is awful to see how far we have fallen. The honey producer claims our government puts certain restrictions and regulations on domestic honey producers that the Chinese do not have to adhere to because of their favored nation status. This man's income has really been slashed and he and the United Airlines employee are facing the same potential health problems.

Several decades ago the State of Illinois produced more food than the entire continent of Africa. This week we ordered some organic vegetables and when we received them they were from China! Thousands of our small farms have gone under because of political decisions. We have forced our small farmer from his land and now we are importing food from around the world. Many of these farmers are still bitter because the farms they lost had been in their families for generations. Our farmers have a right to be upset, but regardless, their health may deteriorate because of it.

Over the last several decades our children have been indoctrinated into a globalization mindset. When they become adults they will not have a clue why there are not any good paying jobs, because those jobs have all been shipped abroad. Out of some 280, 000,000 people living in our country we have less than 15,000,000 producing jobs. How long can these producers carry the entire service industry? If you are one of the fortunate ones who still make a good living in the service industry you will have no interest in someone talking to you about our economic future. Political decisions have been made that created an environment whereby we are eating our children's seed-corn. Any family that is forced to exist without a provider who makes a decent wage is under financial pressure.

Our children are all raised, and we never had the pressure on us that parents have today. This has been brought on for a couple of reasons. Parents are afraid to punish their children for misconduct because of the possibility a state agency may remove the child from their home. States justify the removal on the grounds that the parents are unfit to raise a child. Later when the child grows up, having never been disciplined and never taught to respect their elders, they sometimes commit an unlawful act, and then the state does not make him/her responsible for his/her actions or behavior. When a child is not taught respect for his parents they will not show respect later for a teacher. Our public schools are cesspools mostly because of judicial or political decisions. In America usually both parents work outside of the home. Then parents sometimes feel guilt because of it. If there is a conflict at school with their child the parents will defend the child at all cost. Since the parents are gone for five days a week they will do anything to be a hero to their child. What better way to be a hero to your child than to get them out of trouble? The search for truth is compromised once your primary focus is to play the blame game.

ABC's Good Morning America recently ran a segment on the vast increase of kindergarten children being expelled from school. What a ridiculous state of affairs our public schools have become. When we were kids, any child who acted up was sent to the Principals office who then generated heat in the buttocal area. The procedure was repeated when the child got home! Guess what, the children did not show disrespect to their teachers. The government stopped all of that because this treatment was too inhumane. All you have to do is look at the cesspools that have been created in our public school system and realize what we had years ago was a much more conducive environment for learning. It is no wonder so many children graduate from high school and cannot properly read or write. The point to this is: How much pressure or tension have we put on our children at school? What about those who want to learn? This scenario could be rectified if the government wanted to. Is there a motive for not doing so?

Whether a student graduates or not, if they cannot read or write, you basically send them out in society being ignorant. It is much easier to control someone who is ignorant. I talked to a young college girl who told me one of her classes was teaching how to be in a group and start a discussion to get the group upset. The more people in the group that get upset, and the more disruptive the group gets, the higher the grade the student got. How ridiculous can you be? You merely take a dozen students who do not respect adults and authority, put them in a room together, and you will see disruption!! Parents pay for this education? Colleges and universities have lowered their standards to get more students qualified for enrollment because there is too much government money these schools need to stay open. These institutions have gotten into the business of giving degrees instead of giving educations. This all plays out in a lower level of existence for our country as a whole. Government decisions equate to more stress and tension for all of us. The more stress the government generates equates to a lower quality of life for its citizens, <u>and eventually will play out in the health of the nation.</u>

We have repeatedly pointed out how man is always in the wrong place in his understanding regarding certain subjects. What I am about to share is only done with the intent to show how certain events play out in our health. Our representatives in Washington are spending us into a financial catastrophic situation. Governments will meet their obligations and with debt skyrocketing out of control there is no other option except to inflate the dollar. Now here is the part man has backwards. The masses today are living in a belief system that the currency and inflation are going to be stable and home values are going to escalate. Our current economic environment may temporarily remain the same as it appears today, but the handwriting is on the wall for it to reverse. When it happens our citizens will be financially devastated. Financial situations run in cycles and to be ignorant as to where we are in the cycle can be devastating. If and when a government inflates its currency you have inflation and with it you have higher interest rates. This destroys the housing market which will put even more people out of work and many of those workers will lose their homes. As more homes go on the market the price of existing homes will start to decline. <u>As this scenario plays out it will definitely affect the health of the victims.</u> The train is coming and the masses do not know they are standing on the tracks.

People in the government make mistakes as do all of us. What we do as individuals after we make them will determine the quality of life we have. This holds true for the government as well. A case in point is the dismal failure of the great society initiated by President Johnson back in the 1960's. The more money we pour in the black hole we created only makes the hole deeper. Americans have always been, are now, and will be the most generous people in the world. This is basically because of our Christian heritage. There is however a Christian principle the great society does not adhere to. When a man/woman does not have a job it reflects on the entire community. It is wonderful (it is our duty and responsibility to do so) to give them a helping hand; however, if we do not teach them how to take care of themselves we cripple them. If you give assistance to someone in need, and at the same time you do not teach them how to stand on their own feet and become a contributing member of the community they become crippled. The victims of hurricane Rita do not appear as crippled as those victims of hurricane Katrina. The news media is constantly talking about the expense of Katrina but they are not mentioning Rita near as much. This is mostly because the victims of Rita were in rural areas and these people are for the most part more independent. Rita victims need help to get on their feet but basically they want to fix the problem themselves. Rural people, being more independent, are not looking for as many government handouts. The government punishes independent people by giving more attention to the people in New Orleans. Governments are self-seeking so they reward the inner city people because they are servants of the governmental kingdom. Governments have always worked this way and another perfect example of this is how the news media is showing us how awful the situation is in Africa today. The news released recently is they intend to hit us Americans with a UN tax to help them. The American people will accept this because it is disguised as compassion. In reality it is merely putting the camel's nose under the tent. We all know any money sent to them will always land in the hands of those who are not suffering. The health of citizens in any banana republic is always on the low side and that is exactly the direction we are headed.

Hurricane Katrina attests to the failure mentioned in the above paragraph. It is one thing to have a <u>natural</u> disaster like a hurricane but it is another thing to witness the <u>national</u> disaster that followed. I have read two accounts from volunteers who claimed how awful they were treated trying to assist the victims. Less than 20% of the victims thanked the volunteers for being there for them. One lady said she would not eat that crap when given a MRE (meal ready to eat). I have trouble with that because that is what our servicemen and women eat in the field, while trying to provide for us a free country. The great society has in some cases produced three generations of people on government assistance. When you provide housing, food, education, medical aid to someone you have now created a situation where you cannot give them anything else because they expect it. When the victims did not get what they wanted, when they wanted it, so many of them started acting vulgar to the volunteers. When the victims got <u>angered</u> they compromised their <u>thyroids</u> and the volunteers who were mistreated were put in a position whereby they could have <u>resented</u> the way they were treated. If they did, they compromised their <u>liver</u>. For those ladies who were raped (or were in <u>fear</u> of being raped) after the storm, had their <u>adrenals</u> challenged. Rightfully so! Those acts of violence need to be forgiven because our choices play out in our health one way or the other. Even though the victims must forgive the violators it does not negate the responsibility of our society to arrange for the violators to never be able to repeat it again.

This disaster is a wake up call to all of us, individually and as a country. One lady being interviewed said this was the fourth hurricane she has experienced and it always took four days before help arrived. I am not pointing any fingers but where were the state governments of those gulf coasts states months before the tragedy developed? If all of the citizens along the coast would have had three to four days of water and food stored back, some of the pain might have been lessened. I said in an earlier chapter if we make a mistake we can either justify or rectify it. The mayor of New Orleans did not get his people prepared and instead of apologizing to them he blamed the federal government. *All the people in the government are people so we cannot point fingers at them when they make mistakes; however, if we do not learn from their mistakes we are just as crippled as the victims of the hurricane. If we are expecting the government to take care of us we are blinder than Helen Keller. The news media constantly perpetuates the mindset we need the government to take care of us. We are reeling from all the blunders from Katrina and Rita and now we are faced with a flu epidemic. Two of the main networks were asking the question, "Will the government be ready?"* **I am not free to see my neighbor in need if I am looking for someone to take care of me.**

The only people who get hit and still be able to stand are the ones who are grounded in Him. When Jesus walked here 2000 years ago He was not affected by who ran the politics. He talked to the Roman soldiers and even ministered to them and their families. We must continue our pilgrimage into Him so when a catastrophic situation develops we will not lose our peace. If our security is based on anything man does or does not do, whether in the government or not, then our security is like standing on sand. It is unfortunate most of mankind is standing on sand and political decisions have been made causing so many of our citizens to begin sifting through it. When they realize they are sifting, their health will be compromised. When we put our trust in man we are setting ourselves up for a fall. That is what the masses have done by trusting the government to take care of them. This is why they cannot see the train coming: their false sense of security has blinded them. The health maladies we have pointed out in the earlier chapters await them.

Our founding fathers understood liberty because they understood common law. They understood political power would wipe out the two laws that are essential for a nation to survive, and repeating them: (1) always do what you say you will do, and (2) do not hinder anyone else from their right and freedom to do the same. Everyone living in our country today that has gone through the public school system knows anything about common law. If we lose what little liberty we have left in our nation we are doomed. I point this out merely to say that without liberty you have bondage. If adults do not take responsibility to teach the young the reason we are free, then who will? If we do not understand why we have liberty we will lose it. This is the state of the union today.

As I just said, without liberty you have bondage. Bondage carries with it loads of stress and stress always equates to poorer health. If you know nothing about common law you are part of the problem today in our country. Everyone is looking for someone else to blame for the present conditions we have. If we remain blind to what has happened in our country then we alone are responsible for what we leaving our grandchildren. The stress we are leaving them will for sure affect their quality of life. <u>This includes their health and that of the nation.</u> Again, the only people who will stand upright under the upcoming pressure are the ones grounded in Him. The rest will be buried in the sand and will not have a healthy life.

In the Old Testament God's chosen people were in the wilderness for 40 years. Prior to entering the Promised Land, Moses warned them of what was to come. These people had known bondage their entire lives and now were about to experience liberty and the freedom that comes with it. The warning had to do with handling this new freedom. God's chosen people were chosen to be a beacon light to the rest of the world. God's blessings on them turned them from Him and they took the blessings and became self-absorbed. Prior to Israel becoming a nation no other nation's citizens in history enjoyed the liberty that God's chosen people did. When as a nation they became self-absorbed the nation fell apart. It was 3000 years later that another country enjoyed the same position that Israel of old did, and that is the United States of America. The only thing from history people do not learn is they never learn from it.

In all of recorded history one other nation besides ours enjoyed liberty and freedom and they lost it. We have gone down the same path! The nation of Israel was lost mostly because of David's involvement with Bathsheba and we in our country allowed a President to stay in office for the same offense. God gave us our liberty and we regarded it with contempt. The citizens of Israel were not immediately punished for David's actions but they went into bondage later because of it. Why are we so arrogant that we think the same fate will not happen to us? When He walked with us He looked right in the eyes of the Pharisees and told them they had no eyes to see. We are just as blind as they were and we face the same fate they did. We as a nation have become as self-absorbed and as blind as they were.

Beside the moral issue with Israel I would be remiss if I did not mention another devastating aspect of their culture. God gave them the Ten Commandments to govern their nation. When the lawyers got done they had written over 600 more laws which totally tied the nation in knots. We have allowed the same situation to bind us as well. It has gotten to the point in America you cannot relieve your kidneys unless you are protected by legal council. No wonder lawyers have the only profession condemned in the bible. Luke 11:46, 52 both say, "Woe to you lawyers! Luke 7:30 says, "But the Pharisees and lawyers rejected the will of God for themselves." Is it any wonder why our nation is in such dire straits? The greatest majority of elected officials we send to Washington are lawyers. We have no one to blame but ourselves.

It does not make any difference if you believe this or not, what is developing is coming at a very fast pace. Our own arrogance has blinded us so badly we do not know we are on the track *to destruction. I do not pass judgment on any of our leaders for anything they might have done, but if we do not make them accountable for their actions then we are also guilty of abusing the liberty we have been given.*

One of the main points of this chapter is for us to connect our loss of liberty to our declining health. You will not have optimum health as long as you are in bondage. A case in point is the one who is in financial bondage. How many marriages have failed because of being in financial bondage? Anyone I ever knew who was going through a divorce did not have vibrant health. Regardless of what the bondage may be, it plays itself out in poorer health. Our leaders have guaranteed our nation and its citizens an environment that is conducive to poorer health. *If you read this and do nothing to change the world you live in, you are just as guilty as our leaders.*

There is one vital point I would be remiss if I failed to mention it. The information in this chapter is true and if you look at our nation, in its declining state, we our falling like every other nation before us. Not only did we have Israel as a warning but more recently in our own country we had President Lincoln warn us we would fail within if we were not diligent in protecting our freedom. As history has shown us He was right. In America we have a million dollars worth of intelligence but have a dollars worth of wisdom. Yes, in the natural we are failing but here is the vital point we need to see or we can get depressed real quick. When Columbus landed in America, he and his men knelt down on the beach and dedicated this country to Christ Jesus. The French did the same thing when they landed in the Carolinas, as did the Dutch when they landed in Manhattan, and so did the Pilgrim Fathers on Plymouth Rock. He led His followers to this country, and He helped them conquer it. This country is His because HE paid for it with the blood of His followers. Ps: 33:12 says "Blessed is that nation whose God is the Lord: and the people whom He hath chosen for His own inheritance". He will not allow their blood to be spilled in vain. He will keep this country as it was committed into His hands, but what a price for so many for our disobedience and hardness of heart. The country has walked the way of Cain for so long and it will take catastrophic conditions to restore it. If you are not grounded In Him you are in harm's way.

CONCLUSION

The masses are born and will die in controlled religion, controlled health and controlled politics. When you arrive at the mindset that evil is good then you are controlled. The system has now produced a neutered mind. When that happens to anyone then they now become dependent on the system that wants to destroy all forms of individualism.

I mentioned above we have controlled health. An example of this is reading the chapter on hydrochloric acid and not applying that information to your health regimen. It is amazing how all the commercials for drugs are ended with "ask your doctor." Why should people ask their doctor what they, the patient, might need? Common sense should dictate, because doctors should know what the patient needs. The commercials are a tool to be used as mind control. Most doctors know if they do not write a prescription the patient will go somewhere else to buy it. The pharmaceuticals have mastered the mind control game.

I also mentioned we have controlled religion. If you ask the greatest majority of bible believing Christians if God is in hell, they will adamantly say no. It is amazing how as children we were taught that God is omnipresent (every where), omnipotent (all powerful) and omniscient (all knowing), but they then convince us this is not true. They believe God is everywhere then try to tell us He is not in hell. You cannot have it both ways. If you ask the majority of Christians where did evil come from, they tell you Satan or the devil. They reason a loving God could not make evil. It is simple to find out. Isaiah 45:7 KJV plainly tells us that God made evil. Christians believe something merely because someone told them something and they defend it as the truth. They will tell you God created everything and turn around and tell you Satan created evil. You cannot have it both ways. Most Christian people believe God is going to destroy the earth and bring in a new one. This is merely carnal thinking perpetuated by a carnal thinking system. In Revelation 21:2 it says "and I John saw the Holy City, New Jerusalem, coming down from God out of heaven; prepared as a bride adorned for her husband." So from this verse people think God is going to destroy the earth and bring in another new one. All we have to do is read Rev. 21:5 and God says "I make all things new." I know 2 Peter 3:13 reads, "Nevertheless we, according to His promise, look for new heavens and a new earth in which righteousness dwells." However, if we can see it spiritually we know Peter is talking about people. The earth he mentions is us!! The earth we are, as we are made from dirt. The new heaven is us also. Paul tells us to put on the mind of Christ. The mind of Christ is the new heaven. Only when the Holy Spirit teaches us such things will we be able to read verses with more than the natural mind.

To expound on the above thought I would like to interject something else. I know I have said more than once that man is always standing in the wrong place regarding a particular subject. I will do this one more time before I close. The Holy Spirit is the only one who can teach us The Truth about certain verses. The light (life) we know in the natural comes from the sun. Spiritually Christ Jesus is the Sun of Righteousness. Our earth is decaying all around us and the reason is sin. It is the lack of righteousness (or rightness). When man sinned death entered his world. Paul referred to this as "the law of sin and death" (Rom. 8:2). All of mankind fell into corruption through Adam's disobedience. The scientific name used for this is entropy which means everything in the universe is headed toward decay and disillusionment. About 100 years ago the scientific community formed this into a law called the Second Law of Thermodynamics. This law states that all systems left to themselves become disordered. Entropy controls all things and entropy is nothing other than The Law of Sin and Death. It is amazing to me that Paul told us 2000 years ago this was true and it took man 1900 years to find it out. Man will not believe what God said about the matter but will accept what another man may say and believe it as fact. How long is it going to take man to see the rest of the story? The Almighty God is not going to allow this condition to be permanent. There is a counter-law, a transcendental law, The Law of The Spirit of Life in Christ Jesus. Christ Jesus, the Righteous One, came into the world and was "declared to be the Son of God with power according to the Spirit of holiness" (Rom. 1:4). Can we not see how Holiness is linked to Life and Unrighteousness is linked to Death? The law of entropy (the second law of thermodynamics) can be broken. The Law of Sin and Death can (and will) be superseded. We know this true because Rom. 8:2 says "For the law of the Spirit of life in Christ Jesus has made me free from the law of sin and death." I mentioned earlier that the entire chapter of Romans 8 deals with restoration and man in his carnal nature is still preaching destruction. People still believe what a pastor or priest says, but do not believe what God is saying. The poor flock sits every Sunday looking at the pulpit like a deer starring at the bright lights coming at him. If you are not willing to ask God to do with you what HE did to John the Baptist (mentioned in the next paragraph) then you will be starring at the bright lights for a long time.

John the Baptists' dad was a priest and John would have been a priest automatically; however, God pulled John out of the system and took him out into the wilderness for fourteen years and taught him what He wanted him to know. After that, God sent him back so he could start his ministry. Paul was an educated man and God took him out in the wilderness for the same reason He took John. The point is God knows what we have been taught by our family, friends and schools. He wants to get us alone to teach us what He wants us to know. If this does not happen then we have knowledge within that has been controlled. We must be willing to get out of the box if we are ever going to have more than controlled teaching. Matthew 10:37 says, "He who loves father or mother more than Me is not worthy of Me; and he who loves son or daughter more than Me is not worthy of Me." You can be redeemed and not have this verse a reality in your life, but you will never know Him until it is.

If we are not willing to pay the price to know Him then we will never have abundant life. If we are not willing to apply the natural laws of correct eating in our life, we will not reach our potential either. The same applies to our being willing to have our attitudes changed. When I had cancer I was blessed to have enough people in my life to help me with these three areas of life. The bottom line is that after I applied these principles, I regained my health. There is nothing magical about it. You must be willing to step out of the box and take responsibility for yourself.

We have no control over any thoughts we have but we have total control over what we do with them. When you have a thought a chemical is produced in the brain. Whenever we have a negative or potentially damaging thought we must not try to suppress it or we pay the price for it. You defeat negative thoughts by superceding them with positive thoughts. We are all at times exposed to negative people or situations and unfortunately some people live with them on a daily basis; however, if we have negative thoughts about these people or situations, then we have added another negative to our life. Most people have a mistaken notion thoughts are not important compared to what we say or do. Our thoughts are important because they all play themselves out in what we say or do. It may not play out immediately but eventually it does.

When anyone says or does something that triggers a negative response on our part we should know they have tapped into an unresolved conflict within us. **Our Father always uses these people or circumstances to reveal us to ourselves.** Please read this last sentence again! If you understand it and continue to react negatively when unpleasant circumstances appear, then you still do not see it. After you are able to see it, then our Father starts the process whereby He deals with it. That is why He walks us through the Tabernacle spiritually. Everything travels in threes: (1) He gives us understanding; (2) He gives us eyes to see; (3) He deals with it.

Our thoughts are so important because whether you think you can or cannot, you are right either way. Thoughts are things and things are like gravity, and as you know gravity attracts. This begs the question, "What are your thoughts attracting into your life?" If you are in an unhealthy relationship you certainly cannot blame the other person. **What thoughts did you have that attracted you to them? This same principle applies to our health. When we lose our health we must ask ourselves what thoughts we had that attracted this particular disease. If we will not do this we are left only with the option of having someone else deal with our symptoms.**

We recently had the opportunity to visit several Scandinavian countries and we were in awe of the beauty there. More important though, I saw something in myself I had never seen before. When we were in Finland we learned in the last century they were in bondage to the Swedes, the Germans and the Russians at various times. Being able to see enemy soldiers in your country is an obvious bondage. The thing I learned about myself was that at the same time their bondage was going on I was in the United States completely oblivious to what was going on over there. In high school here life seemed to be good. We went to school, got a job after school for spending money and had no thoughts that life would not always be good. Later, after getting married, things started to fall apart.

You start to feel that darkness will overtake you, but in reality the opposite was true. The darkness that I was experiencing was really a tool to expose the darkness that was always there within me. Jeremiah 17:9 says, "The heart is deceitful above all things." This sure was me because those people over there knew they were in bondage but I was blind to mine. We may live in a free country but this cannot make us free from ourselves. I asked myself who had been in the most bondage, those people in Finland or me? I had to admit it was me. Man may allow us freedom on the outside but only Christ Jesus can make us free within. Very few people live at this level of freedom.

People for centuries have tried to ignore, deny, suppress or try to escape the reality of the above verse in Jeremiah but to no avail. Man in his carnal nature feels if you do not deal with the depravity of the heart it will eventually go away. It never does! The reality of man's sin has filled our mental hospitals and prisons to the brink. The majority of the people in our mental hospitals are there primarily because their lives are overwhelmed by their sin which they have done their best to ignore. Prior to these people being made zombies in our mental facilities, by all the medication they have been given, there was a solution for the greatest majority of them. If someone would have shown them these four verses:(Ps 32:2, Rom 4:8, 1 Cor 1:30, Col 1:21-22) and explained the magnitude of these verses to them, most of them would not have ended up where they are today. If the majority of the rest of them would have been given something to stabilize their blood sugar and given ample amounts of B-vitamins, with emphasis on B-12, there would not have been enough patients left to keep these institutions open. This is merely another example of understanding the importance of dealing with the person and not just the body.

In chapter one I stated we were created spirit (Gen. 1:26), and in Genesis 2:7 it says, "and man became a living soul." The word became is a progressive action verb. So man became something he had not been. I prefaced this book on the fact that we are spirit, soul and body. I did that because this is the reality most of Christendom lives in today, but the truth is much more than this. We mentioned earlier the marriage feast of The Lamb was a marriage within. Our soul is to become submissive to the spirit until the two become one. At that point we will be spirit and body. When this happens we will have experienced our own ascension the same as He did. When we come to realize He is The Truth and everything outside of Him in the universe is not, then we know everything outside of Him that people believe, is fabricated in or from the mind of man. When we become conscious of this, we will know we have squandered our true inheritance, which is our life in Him or life abundant. When we become conscious of this we then realize we have lived life as the <u>prodigal son</u>.

Prayer is essential, but I always tell people you are wasting your time praying for something when His answer is already in His word. An example of this is when Moses started praying on the shore and God told him to get up and put his foot in the water. He has instructed us about our attitudes. It is our responsibility to do what we are told to do by our Father. If we do not, we are standing on sand. We cannot do what He tells us to do until He makes us free. Young people think they can move away from their parents and be free, but this is wishful thinking. Freedom is not being able to do what you want to do; it is <u>being free to do what is right</u>. True freedom enables us to live in His joy and until we do we will continue to fight the battle of Armageddon (the battle we all have to fight until the roaring lion within is defeated).

<u>If everyone and every government would adhere to the two principles that ensure human liberty: (A) always do what you say you will do, and (B) never infringe on the rights of others so they are free to do the same, we would have peace. Keep in mind that peace is more than the absence of strife or trouble, but a state of mind going through the trials and tribulations of life. That is the essence of this entire book, how to have peace within. If we do not, the best food we may consume will not give us vibrant health. Lack of peace affects us whether individually or corporately as a nation.</u>

May God bless you as you put your foot in the water as Moses did! Water in this case represents your problems, whether they are spiritual, emotional or physical.

I want to conclude with one of my favorite bible stories. 2 Sam. 9:1-13 records the story of King David wanting to show kindness to someone in Saul's house because of the love David had for Saul's son Jonathan. They found Jonathan's son and his name was Mephibosheth. David's servants told him the son was crippled in both feet. David had the boy summoned. Now try putting yourself in the young man's place. What would you think if you were poor and crippled and the King's men show up saying the King called for you? Mephibosheth had to be scared because it says he prostrated himself before the king. People today go nuts when they win a million dollars and this is nothing compared to what David gave him. The king gave him all the land his grandfather Saul had plus the grandson got to eat at the King's table for life. Today one can squander their winnings and end up paupers, but here he lived the life of royalty forever. Today Our Father is calling us to His table to eat with Him forever. He is calling everyone who is deformed physically, mentally and emotionally devastated. **In the natural people pay for bread and they are fed crumbs, but spiritually people have been led to believe they only deserve crumbs and our Father is offering them the whole loaf, The Bread of Life.**

It has been a privilege to share part of my life and part of my heart with you.

RECOMMENDED READING

In reference to health, there are monthly publications I have subscribed to for years. These men and their staffs have dedicated themselves to helping mankind have a better quality of life. Many people have asked me in the past where I learned a particular thought, and I can honestly tell them I do not know. When you read numerous publications monthly it is impossible over time to remember where you learned it all. That is why I am listing them so credit may go where it deserves. If you are unfamiliar with these publications, I would highly recommend them.

Alternatives:

www.drdavidwilliams.com
1-800-887-8262

Dr. Julian Whitaker's
Health & Healing
1-888-886-8213

Dr. William Campbell Douglass's
Real Health Breakthroughs
1-800-851-7100

The Bob Livingston Letter
P.O. Box 110013
Birmingham, Al. 35211
1-800-773-5699

The High Blood Pressure Hoax
by Sherry A. Rogers, M.D.

For more detailed spiritual insight as to the tabernacle Moses built I would highly recommend two publications.

The Key to the Priesthood
David Ebaugh Bible School
102 Park Terrace
Harrisburg, Pa. 17111

Kingdom Bible Studies
J. Preston Eby
P. O. Box 371240
El Paso, Tx. 79937-1240
Ask for the Royal Priesthood Series

A book I found very helpful in showing the difference between the spirit and the soul is:

The Third Salvation
David Ebaugh Bible School
102 Park Terrace
Harrisburg, Pa. 17111

Two books I have recommended to my customers for those suffering from adrenal exhaustion are as follows:

From Fatigued to Fantastic
By Jacob Teitelbaum, M. D.

Adrenal Fatigue
By James L. Wilson, N.D., D.C., Ph.D

A good book for understanding what is best for us to eat:

Eat Right 4 Your Type
By Dr. Peter J. D'Adamo

We mentioned earlier Christian people have been taught fables and for those who are serious about their walk then I highly recommend:

Read and Search God's Plan
By Dr. Harold Lovelace
P.O. Box 995
Saraland, Al. 36571
www.HaroldLovelace.com
godallinall@juno.com

If you would ike to contact us via the web or mail:

www.shaneblackburn.com
Shane Blackburn
P.O. Box 95, Hicksville, Ohio
43526